CURED
by NATURE

CURED
by NATURE

HOW TO HEAL FROM THE INSIDE OUT, FIND HAPPINESS, AND DISCOVER YOUR TRUE SELF

TARA MACKEY

FOREWORDS BY TODD COOPER & JOSH ROSEBROOK

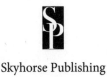

Skyhorse Publishing

Skyhorse Publishing books may be purchased in bulk at special discounts for sales promotion, corporate gifts, fund-raising, or educational purposes. Special editions can also be created to specifications. For details, contact the Special Sales Department, Skyhorse Publishing, 307 West 36th Street, 11th Floor, New York, NY 10018 or info@skyhorsepublishing.com.

Skyhorse® and Skyhorse Publishing® are registered trademarks of Skyhorse Publishing, Inc.®, a Delaware corporation.

Visit our website at www.skyhorsepublishing.com.

10 9 8 7 6 5 4 3 2 1

Library of Congress Cataloging-in-Publication Data

Names: Mackey, Tara, 1986-author.
Title: Cured by nature : how to heal from the inside out, find happiness,
    and discover your true self / Tara Mackey.
Description: New York, NY : Skyhorse Publishing, [2016]
Identifiers: LCCN 2015037362 | ISBN 9781634504010 (hardcover : alk. paper)
Subjects: LCSH: Mackey, Tara, 1986- | Naturopathy. | Nature, Healing power
    of. | Alternative medicine. | Well-being.
Classification: LCC RZ440 .M3335 2016 | DDC 615.5/35—dc23
LC record available at http://lccn.loc.gov/2015037362

Cover design by Erin Seaward-Hiatt
Cover photo credit: The Organic Life, LLC

Print ISBN: 978-1-63450-401-0
Ebook ISBN: 978-1-63450-884-1

Printed in the United States of America

CONTENTS

• • • • • • • •

FOREWORD BY TODD COOPER   vii
FOREWORD BY JOSH ROSEBROOK   ix
INTRODUCTION   xi

PART ONE: BE HAPPY   1

CHAPTER ONE
Why You Want to Be Happy, but Aren't (and How to Start)   2

CHAPTER TWO
Breath: The Universal Healer   37

CHAPTER THREE
The Breakthrough   65

CHAPTER FOUR
My Name Is Herb   79

PART TWO: STAY WEIRD   115

CHAPTER FIVE
The Dream   116

CHAPTER SIX
How to Create Lasting Change   146

CHAPTER SEVEN
The Time You Have   167

CHAPTER EIGHT
Wisdom: The Greatest Cleanser   185

PART THREE: LIVE WELL   203

CHAPTER NINE
Green Beauty   204

CHAPTER TEN
The Teacher Appears   240

CHAPTER ELEVEN
Daily Miracles   257

CHAPTER TWELVE
Lifelong Healing   287

NOTES   309

For My Family
<3

"The Earth supplies me with everything I need."
—Paramahansa Yogananda (1893–1952),
Indian Yogi and Guru, Author,
Founder of the Self-Realization Fellowship,
Cosmic Man

FOREWORD
by Todd Cooper

It was during a trip back to New York that Tara got the email. "They want me to write a book!" she told me. "Who is 'they,'" I asked, "and what kind of book?"

Tara said the editors at Skyhorse Publishing in New York City had been following her blog and had offered her a book deal. "You HAVE to write a book! The world needs to know about your experiences!" they had said.

This is very rare, but it is not a fluke. Tara is almost always reading, researching, creating, or writing. She told me that some of her best friends from high school were the music teacher and the librarian. While doing research, I saw her get so excited about a book that she read all six hundred pages and returned it to the library the day after she checked it out.

Everything about this experience has been serendipitous for Tara. This book was meant to be; this story has to be told. Everyone needs to read *Cured by Nature*. It smashes conventional misconceptions about personal health, and it will change your life.

Three months is not a lot of time to write a three-hundred-page book, especially if you already work full-time. It has taken me quite a long time to write this very short foreword. But three months' time is exactly how long it took Tara to start—and finish—her first draft of *Cured by Nature*. During those months she had a role in a feature film and was on set for over a month of that time. She was in a few major music videos, wrote blog posts, made ads for brands, and still managed to carve out more than forty hours a week to research and write.

At times Tara would tell me that it was like the book was writing itself. There were days she would say she could hardly even remember writing it, but that it all felt perfect. After a few tweaks, Tara produced an amazing, one-of-a-kind, must-read, inspirational, timeless classic.

Tara was living her life as she was writing about it, so the process was all encompassing. Her story is so real and so familiar that everyone needs to hear it. However dramatic and daring Tara's life has been, everyone can relate to it in some way. All of the subject matter is so current and relevant that you can almost taste it. It's empowering and enthralling. No book has changed my life more.

I hope *Cured by Nature* revolutionizes your life the way it has changed mine.

Todd Cooper
CEO of Waxelene, Inc.

FOREWORD
by Josh Rosebrook

The clean beauty and wellness community is a collective of empowered, empathetic individuals. We are a tribe. We are beauty experts and professionals who've connected through a shared passion and vision for clean cosmetics, natural foods, and conscious, holistic lifestyle.

This tribe of natural beauty experts is truly special and includes writers, entrepreneurs, practitioners, and artists. I'm honored to be a part of it, and I'm continually amazed by the breadth of integrity, sensitivity, knowledge, and action each person brings to the collective. Whether we meet up with each other online or at a workshop, event, or conference, we corroborate, support, and empathize with each other steadfastly, which is the ultimate healing. Within this connected experience, there's an authentic framework that is built, and everyone inspires and supports each other. This type of real community is what we all need to manifest our dreams and passions and find or stay on our true path.

I became aware of Tara through our community, and one day I found myself on her website theorganiclifeblog.com. I was intrigued by her writing style. Her words seemed effortlessly executed and her authenticity drew me in. Her narrative revealed someone who was extremely confident, connected, and self-aware. I knew I liked her.

There weren't many fellow "green beauties" (as we like to call them) living in Los Angeles at the time, so once we realized we were both Angelenos, we knew we had to meet.

On a sunny Sunday during the winter in LA we met up at Real Food Daily. It was one of those rare friendships that seemingly comes out of nowhere: you have a feeling that you've known this person before and you connect non-stop for three hours over tempeh and tea. It was glorious. She exuded the genuine joy, humor, and heart that makes everyone feel special. Today, I am honored to call her one of my great friends.

Cured by Nature is not just another guide on how to live naturally or telling you what makeup and skin-care products you should purchase; it's much more than that. This book contains a vibration that has the potential to shift you emotionally, mentally, spiritually, and physically — if you are ready. This book was created with a grand intention to assist humanity in waking up to whatever might be keeping you down in any way. Whether it's the food you eat or your relationship to it, the toxic beauty products you still use, your intimate relationships that are stuck, or whatever disconnected voice of fear that might be running through your head that needs to be released, *Cured by Nature* carries a vibration of Light and Love that calls us to take full responsibility for who we are and to integrate real, positive change while nudging us to remember that we are incredibly brilliant, divine, powerful human beings who can do, be, and have anything.

Thank you, Tara, for imbuing my life with such truth, clarity, and action via this book. You are a pioneer of healing for a generation and a leader for anyone ready to be inspired, grow, and make changes.

Josh Rosebrook
Founder, Josh Rosebrook Skin and Hair Care

INTRODUCTION

My mother was an Irish immigrant in the midst of achieving the American Dream. She was beautiful—a bold, bodacious, curvaceous redhead who had even earned a great modeling gig in the monthly business magazine from her Wall Street employer in New York City. She was the talk of the staff elevator rides and the envy of all her co-workers. Her steady boyfriend of seventeen years idolized and adored her, showed her off to all his friends. He bought her cars and puppies and extravagant gifts. They partied—a lot.

But they had been having problems. Relationship issues. Bitter fights. She was taking days off from work to figure things out. Hitting up bars with her girlfriends, staying out later than she always expected. The night she and her boyfriend broke up for good, she stumbled into a bar she'd never been to before.

There, a man asked her for the time. She looked down to check her watch, but before she could answer, a young, buff, surly stranger with piercing green eyes decked the other guy across the face. The provocateur grabbed her arm and began to run, shouting, "Let's get out of here! This is my uncle's place! I shouldn't have done that!"

A whirlwind romance ensued. She found out the stranger's name: Dan. And his occupation: Queens' dirtiest drug dealer. Still, she couldn't help but think he was handsome, attractive, and confident. Every block they walked down, someone shouted Dan's name in friendly recognition. He had the gift of gab and a strong hustle. She fell for him—hard. He was twenty-seven. She was twenty-nine. Perfect.

At seven months pregnant, all these thoughts are inescapable. What led her here? Locked in a dark room in a dingy Queens apartment while Dan, his goons, and his other girls talk outside the door. It turns out that Dan is nineteen—not twenty-seven as he'd claimed—and she's seen him about as much as she's *not* seen him. Her secure job is long gone. He keeps her in the bedroom and locks the door from the outside. He cooks crack instead of dinner. He feeds her drugs when he remembers.

When labor comes, she's alone. Dan's been gone for days. A cab takes her to the hospital where she informs doctors that she's giving birth—and high. They knock her out and cut the baby out of her. The baby is sent straight to NICU for detox.

Days later, Dan comes home to an empty house. Suspecting the obvious, he finds the hospital his girl's at, and he tries to see her. He confidently strolls down the halls of the hospital, swagger-drunk, congratulating himself on his new baby boy to nurses and strangers.

When he enters the hospital room, she screams and screams until nurses come and tell Dan he has to leave. She continues screaming as he's dragged away.

"Get the fuck out of here!" she yells after him. "You're not welcome here! *You'll have absolutely nothing to do with my daughter's life!*"

My biological father's information on my birth certificate is completely blank. I have my mother's last name—Mackey—and the name that *Dad*, my Irish maternal grandfather, picked out for me—Tara. My mother said she never even thought about what to name me until she held me in her arms.

It would be two weeks in detox for me and another seven years before my biological parents would see each other again. When my mother said my biological father would have absolutely nothing to do with my life, she meant it.

PART ONE:
BE HAPPY

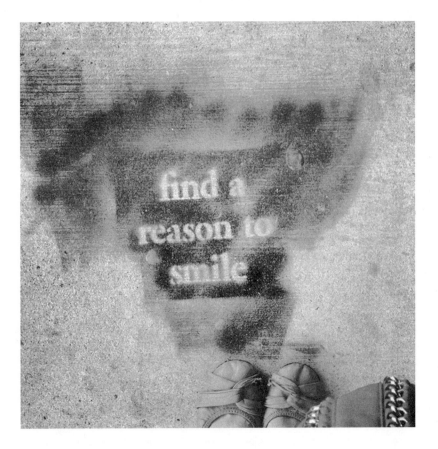

CHAPTER ONE

WHY YOU WANT TO BE HAPPY, BUT AREN'T (AND HOW TO START)

"You won't be happy, whatever you do, unless you're comfortable in your own conscience. Keep your head up, keep your shoulders back, keep your self-respect, be nice, be smart. And remember: there are practically no 'overnight' successes."

—Lucille Ball (1911–1989),
Actress, Comedian, Entrepreneurial TV Badass

Organic Life

At six years old, I couldn't wake my mom up. She was lying in bed barely breathing. I pulled her eyelids back from her eyes; they were stark white. So I got a chair from the dining room, stood on it to reach the phone, and called my grandparents.

My sweet Irish grandpa, whom we affectionately call Dad, showed up and whisked me into a car where I stayed, locked and helpless, while ambulances came. That was the last, but not the first, time I saw my mom overdose on heroin, and within a few weeks I was in a private, backdoor courtroom, testifying against her at my custody hearing, while a stenographer typed away.

By the age of seven, I had witnessed more than most adults I knew, and felt different as a result. Moreover, I knew that I might always feel and might possibly always *be* different. That thought alone was daunting and depressing. My mom was in and out of rehab, always promising to "get me back" and then disappearing for weeks on end. I spent many long nights imagining worst-case scenarios, like having to attend her funeral.

This started a serious case of childhood insomnia. In photos from ages seven through ten I look downright sickly—some days the bags under my eyes almost reached my cheekbones. I couldn't sleep for anything. Figuring out how I was going to explain my living situation to friends was troubling to me as well. I cared an awful lot about what other people thought, and was always conscious of what I said around them.

It was also around this age that my maternal grandparents received custody of me, becoming my legal guardians. Grandma and Dad were absolutely the most amazing parents a little girl could ask for. Grandma is a sweet, beautiful soul with a thick Irish accent. Even though she can only boast a seventh-grade education, she's hands-down the most intelligent and insightful woman I know. Dad's accent remained equally adorable and slathered on like he just stepped off the boat. Underneath it Dad embodied a quiet, understanding, and loving father figure. Although the word "love" rarely left their mouths, they showed it in every way they could think of. They were hell-bent on providing me with everything I could possibly need, and especially determined that I not turn out anything like my mother.

They had been done raising their own children years ago, and here I was: helpless, wild, and in need of their care. They were in their mid-fifties, and had a brand-new kid.

Inherently Different

When you're a child of an addict, life is just inherently different. A lot of people spend a lot of time trying to convince you that the addict's behavior is *not* your fault, that you are *not* the trigger. I did believe this, deep down. I knew that if I didn't have the power to make my mom stop drinking (and I didn't), I certainly didn't have the power to make my mom drink.

I may not have been the reason my mom drank or did drugs, but I was certainly never the most savory topic of conversation. As the years wore on, it seemed as though I was the source of every fight, every contention, and every source of malice within my family. "What are we going to do with her?" and "She's going to grow up just like her mother!" rang throughout my house more times as a child than I can count for even the smallest of infractions. They may not have said it right in front of me, but that doesn't mean I didn't hear it.

I get it. They were scared to death that I was going to end up like my mom. But at the time, I was clueless about how to handle myself. Every small contention turned into an outburst. Every outburst, a fight. Every fight, a panic attack.

I threw a few temper tantrums when I started living with my grandparents full-time. I've heard a couple of less-than-pretty stories from my neighbors about me screaming in the driveway that I wasn't going anywhere and that I wanted my mom. But I quickly caught on.

The life spent waiting in hot cars or stairwells while my mom "saw friends," going to the gas station alone with only a note to pick up cigarettes for her at four and five years old, or wondering if she was going to be awake in the morning was gone.

I was sent to talk therapy the same month I started living with my grandparents full-time. I was very melancholy and super precocious, and I found a lot of comfort in this sadness. I wore my life story like a badge of honor and my therapist, an amazing man named Dr. Dial, encouraged me to talk about it extensively, and to whomever I wished.

This helped me tremendously in my recovery and encouraged a healthy and honest way to cope with my emotions, even to this day. I have never been ashamed that my story was different, and I have always been eager to share it. Through sharing my life story I have even learned that many people have gone through similar situations, strayed down similar paths, and come out on similar sides. But as a kid, that never stopped me from *wishing it was less difficult.*

With my grandparents as my parents, I finally took regular showers, finally ate a meal at the table every night, finally didn't have to share a room with anyone, and finally didn't have to do everything myself. That was the hardest adjustment. I still prefer to do things myself: this may take a few more decades to wear off.

A whirlwind of ambulances (for Mom), Alateen support groups (for me and the other children of alcoholics in the neighborhood), and alienation among friends made the next few years difficult emotionally. I was super grateful to have my grandparents in my life, and I adjusted to my living situation pretty well, but I still had a lack of social skills that was really interfering with my life.

Bathing every day, for example, was a new concept to me. So was not being able to do whatever I wanted with no supervision. I wasn't used to adults hovering over me and didn't like it one bit. I remember my grandma telling me once, "You realize one time we found you with your hand in your mother's purse, holding onto a razor and drugs, when you were three years old! Three!"

I had seen a lot worse than some razors or a bag of drugs, but I got it; I knew my grandparents were concerned. I wanted to change and I wanted to be better. I just *didn't know how*. It felt as though someone were trying to whip the spirit out of me instead of guiding me along my own path.

When I was seven, my uncle, who was eager to help, gave me two presents that both changed my life forever and helped me cope with my problems. One was the book *Awaken the Giant Within* by motivational speaker and life coach Anthony Robbins and the second was a set of various audiotapes for *Unleash the Power Within* (also by Tony). I listened to these tapes day after day after day for years, and read this book over and over again, underlining what I understood and dog-earing what I knew I would understand "when I get older."

Repeatedly listening to these tapes and catching *Oprah* at 4 p.m. with Grandma every day after school put my problems in perspective. I had a vague idea, both from caring for my mom and from watching shows like *Oprah* and listening to people like

Tony, that life did not get easier when you got older. It didn't get easier and you needed to know how to handle it. I was determined to learn how to make a better life for myself than what I had seen happen to people around me.

Saying Yes

When I was seven a cute little kitten walked into my aunt's yard during a party over the summer and would not leave my side. I begged my grandparents to let us take him home, and finally, my grandma said yes!

We named the black-and-white bubba Sylvester, but a few weeks later, after his first checkup, we were informed that Sylvester was, unfortunately for our name choice, a girl.

Miss Sylvester, or Sylvia, was a staple in my household well into college. Moving in with my grandparents had been a huge transition for me, and having an animal I doted on, called my own, and loved with everything in me was the best kind of therapy. Sylvia followed me to school, accompanied Pebbles the dog, Dad, and me on nightly walks, and cuddled with me at night before I fell asleep. She was the subject of every creative paper I wrote and every doodle I drew. She provided comfort in times when everyone else had no idea what to do with me.

Tentatively Thrilled

Kindergarten to sixth grade is a blur of plaid skirts, play auditions, voice lessons, dog walks with Dad, long hours rehearsing for Mass at the church across the street, Jesus statues, the best musical theater experiences of my life, and a lot of personal growth.

I accepted my living situation gracefully. Although, with two generations between my grandparents and me, there was bound to sometimes be contention, I loved them both deeply. I knew I would have absolutely no life without them, and often cried softly at night, scared to lose them. Scared they'd suddenly decide they didn't love me. Scared, knowing they'd die before all my friends' parents did. Scared, knowing they'd chosen me and might ultimately decide they'd made a mistake. Scared everyone would decide not to love me. I worried a lot about things like being abandoned, being helpless, or losing someone that I loved.

When I was eleven, my mom finally sobered up. She spent over a year at a rehab center and when she was done my grandparents tried one last tactic: let her live with us and be the mother she was always begging them to let her be.

I was tentatively thrilled. Just four years after they had gained temporary custody, there was a glimmer of hope: Mom might actually step up to the plate and get me back. She worked her program, made lots of friends in sobriety, and really lived what she was preaching.

Before long she even became someone else's sponsor, leading meetings and helping others recover. She once told me that just looking down the beer aisle at the grocery store made her nauseous. It was a really lovely time in my life. It felt like I had a family, and I took a lot of pride in my new family dynamic. I now had **three** parents—beat *that*!

My mother and I were as close as ever. She was dating someone who had been sober for fifteen years and loved her and me a lot. We all trusted one another.

Too Weird

Then came adolescence. I had a great clique of three girlfriends in sixth grade, and then suddenly, without explanation, they all decided I was "too weird" to hang out with. They decided I didn't fit in with them. This group of girls did things like invite me to their houses, then sit inside and laugh as I rang the doorbell, never welcoming me in. They'd steal my lunch box and throw it around to one another until my lunch was ruined. They'd ignore me if I spoke to any of them in class. I was astounded; I'd never experienced anything like this before!

Then, they started making fun of the way I looked. I was the only mixed girl in my entire school—half Irish on my mom's side and black and Native American on my biological father's—and was told almost every day in less and less nice ways that I was not the prettiest person to look at.

This was alarming to me, not only because I had never even thought twice about my own appearance (or anyone else's) and put no effort into it at all, but also because I personally didn't hate looking at myself! I didn't understand what the big deal was. At all. I was also astounded that there was no way to "go back" to the way things used to be in our friendships. They were *over* me.

On top of this, I was socially awkward, thin as a rail, tall, gangly, relatively serious, clumsy, and really embarrassing in gym class. Basically, I was a bully's dream come true. Sometimes I was made fun of for being a teacher's pet, or not being as affluent as the other kids I went to school with, which continued well into college. It was everything I had feared, and it was relentless no matter what school I went to or what kinds of friends I made.

Normal Life

The summer before I was to start high school, Grandma, Dad, Mom, and I took a vacation to Florida. I still treasure the pictures from that time. The four of us look so happy, so healthy. My mom has a glowing tan and her arm embraces me with pride in every photo.

My mother happily lived a sober life with my grandparents and me for two solid years. She really was stepping up to the plate, making up for lost time in the form of NYC outings, weekly dinners out, and support in all my creative endeavors. She started taking college classes, had a great, new job nursing, and was even beginning to save for things like voice lessons and college for me. I was getting a small glimpse of what a normal life might be like. Our family was as close as ever, and I was finally beginning to believe that I could soon drop the "inherently different" label. It was clear that sobriety was most important to my mother. More than drugs, more than drinking, and more than dependent relationships, she wanted to be well. My grandparents felt so comfortable that they went on vacation together and left me and mom to watch the house.

Within a few days of their departure, there were telltale signs that I couldn't ignore. They felt and looked all too familiar. My mom was spending a lot of time alone, or out with a young girl whose sponsor she had just become. Then, she started smoking in the house, falling asleep in the middle of the day, and leaving big cigarette burns in the bedsheets. Her words were more slurred, her temper became nastier, and she was starting to avoid being around me.

Finally, I found it. A bottle of vodka hidden under her bed in my childhood playroom, which I had given up so my mom could have a bedroom. I told my grandparents the moment they came home from vacation and waited for the shit storm. It came in one large drove.

One of my last memories of that time is my mother clinging onto the doorframe as my grandpa pulled her out the door by her legs. She was lying there crying and trying to explain why she's drunk, screaming, "Help me, Tara! Help me!"

I went over to the door, looked at her, looked down at her fingers, stared her straight in the face, and kicked her fingers over and over again as hard as I could until she let go. Somehow, they managed to get her into the car and off to the hospital. After that, I didn't see her again for a few years.

I like to think I did help.

Feeling Different

This time, I was emotionally done with her. It was the first time I had deeply felt this *done*-ness, and it stole a part of my heart. However, it felt absolutely necessary at the time. When she was in rehab, my grandpa constantly encouraged me to talk to my mom, but I just couldn't do it. There was nothing left in it for me. I knew what a bad influence looked like, even when it was my parent.

I was thirteen and about to start at an all-girls Catholic high school. It was not my favorite—I would have preferred the co-ed theater-driven Catholic school—but it was the best there was, and I'd gotten in, so it was there I went.

In the back of my mind I was very fearful that any amount of love or trust I showed anyone would be betrayed or taken away at the first opportunity. This is a fear that I remember feeling very, very early. A fear that developed into anxiety as I grew older. Whether it was this anxiety, fear, hormones, or just being a teenager, I finally told my grandma one night that I "felt different."

Sharing this prompted a fear in her to do something she hadn't, to my knowledge, done before. She read my diaries while I was at school, which I'd kept since the age of seven. They were full of angry, self-hating, family-mistrusting rants for page after tear-stained page. Grandma sat me down about this, but I had no explanation. I meant every single word that I had written, and furthermore I now felt very betrayed by *her* actions as well as my mom's. In fact, I considered never writing again. I was becoming more and more bitter about life and people by the day.

I was pretty broody, and a little boy- (and girl-) crazy, but I wasn't really turning out to be the drug-fiending, "rehab is my second home," skip-town misfit that my family always feared I would be. In fact, I was astonishingly polite, loved learning, and (mostly) knew when to be quiet. I sang at multiple Masses at church every Sunday, got First Honors every semester, read books for fun, and enjoyed time alone in the dirt and at the library. I mean, it could have (and had) been way worse for them. However, out of a combination of fear and love, I was still treated as a ticking time bomb and a potential fuck-up.

Lithium

I crept to the staircase after my bedtime and listened quietly. On the top step I was just out of sight. While holding my breath, I heard almost every word of the heated debate about what to do with me. It was finally decided that I should stop talk therapy with my beloved Dr. Dial and be sent to a psychiatrist for "evaluation."

I wordlessly went to the appointment, although I had no idea what the difference was between this new doctor and my old one. I thought I was going to another therapist to talk about my life, my feelings, and my problems. I thought I was going to a more qualified person to work through the newest curveballs life had thrown my way.

After a half-hour discussion with my grandma, and a five-minute "interview" that consisted of no more than ten questions for me, my new doctor—a child psychiatrist—diagnosed me with bipolar II, or manic depressive disorder.

This was a diagnosis that I was actually familiar with, even at that age—a close relative had bipolar disorder. His life, according to my grandmother, had "been ruined" because of it, and he had been on medication for as long as I could remember. Other family members had also been diagnosed with emotional disorders too.

My biological father was never a part of my childhood—my mother made sure of it—and I never asked about him. Not once. But I did hear one story: his mother—my grandmother—had been schizophrenic, and she committed suicide in front of him when he was young. This had definitely been relayed to my psychiatrist. It may have been everything he needed to know.

At thirteen, I was dealing pretty well with everything happening in my life. Sure, I was emotionally unstable, confused, hormonal, and preferred long hours of reading or video games to social activities with people who might ask about my life, but it was also my first year as a teenager, and I felt okay despite the fact that my mom had relapsed in front of me (again). All in all, whether my diagnosis from the psychiatrist was a preemptive strike based on family history, or whether this doctor actually thought that the bitter, inquisitive, and hopeful thirteen-year-old in front of him with a terrible backstory was truly mentally ill, I might never know.

Dr. Brown explained that what I had was very serious, and said that without medication I would never "live a normal life."

He put me on lithium, a powerful sedative first prescribed in the 1800s for "hysteria"—500 mg a day, even though I was *maybe* eighty-five pounds at the time. I was told, not once or twice, but every time I saw Dr. Brown, and just about every day at home, that I could never stop taking this medication, even when I felt better.

In fact, every single time I ever told Dr. Brown that I wanted to come off lithium, either because it made me feel better **or** worse, he would say that wanting to stop my medication was a very serious symptom of the illness, and sometimes even increased my dosage. This medical catch-22 was infuriating to me because I hated that stuff from day one . . .

"Happiness cannot be traveled to, owned, earned, worn, or consumed."

—Denis Waitley (1933–Present),
Motivational Speaker, Author, Founding Member of the
National Council for Self-Esteem, Success Guru

And this is where my story really begins: the first year that I gave my life over to medication, the first year I let someone else convince me that I was powerless over my emotions, and that a pill was there to solve my problems. Because, let's face it, with a story like mine, that thirteen-year-old girl does seem pretty powerless, doesn't she?

YOUR PERCEPTION

I talk to her. I often talk to thirteen-year-old me and tell her who she is going to become. I tell her that she's beautiful and capable and hysterical and adventurous and spiritual and talented and loved. I tell her to cherish the family dinners, to scale back her anger, to think before she speaks, and to hug her family every day even if they don't want her to.

Recently a mentor asked me a question that his mentor had asked him.

"Who's going to take care of seventy-year-old you, Tara?"

"I don't know." I meditated on it for a moment, but I'd actually, literally, never thought about it. I tried to reply, "My kids, probably? My family?"

"The only person who's going to take care of seventy-year-old you is you *right now*."

That struck me very hard. I realized that this "talking to myself" could be done two ways: in addition to talking to my past self, I could also talk to my present, as seventy-year-old me.

I constantly started telling myself to make healthier, more meaningful, and attractive decisions. I started taking risks I wouldn't normally take. I actively sought out every sunset and I deliberately stopped to smell every flower. I drove down every coast. I made it a goal to get to the top of every mountain. *Why?*

Well, because I want seventy-year-old Tara to be proud of me, the way that Tara today is proud of thirteen-year-old Tara. I have thought about that philosophy and shaped my life around it every day since. It has positively formed how I care for my body, my mind, and what I allow to become part of my life philosophy.

The best thing that I can do now is talk to twenty-something-year-old me *as* seventy-year-old me, which I actually do very often. I talk to myself now, as my future self. Seriously. I tell myself I got this, that what I'm doing is easy, that I can handle things, and that nothing that I've ever done is in vain. I tell myself I'm capable and beautiful and smart and super awesome, and I believe it. I always hope that future me believes it too.

"At any given moment, life is completely senseless. But over a period, it seems to reveal itself into an organism existing in time, having a purpose, tending in a certain direction."

—Aldous Huxley, Prolific Author,
Philosopher, Trip Enthusiast

You are **not** your backstory. Your story has essentially been what you've told yourself. When I was telling myself "I am not like other people" or "I am not worthy of happiness" every day, my unworthy feeling was based on nothing but my past. My *present notion* of *who I used to be* determined **everything**. I felt unworthy because I was not as rich or as beautiful, because I never had the same nuclear family dynamic other people had. Whatever it was, I was creating a story based entirely on my perception, and my past beliefs. Since our beliefs are nothing *but* perceptions, this cycle can be endless.

Perception is a mirror. It is your present notion of yourself and your world, reflected outward. Your life is, indeed, organic. It grows and changes with every breath. Perception is the outward reflection of the greatest tool we have for changing our whole lives.

Beliefs

We are very often seduced into believing that events control our lives, or that we are powerless to our past. Nothing can be further from the truth. A belief is a feeling of certainty about something or someone. If you say, "I believe I can climb that mountain," all you're really saying is that you have a strong **emotional certainty** that you're capable of climbing that mountain. Really, it's not even entirely important if the beliefs you hold *are true*. What matters most is whether or not your beliefs **empower your life** or limit your life.

Our Limiting Beliefs

Thoughts like: "I hate where I live or work," "I'm stuck here," "I'm stifled in this place," "I need a pill to get through this day," and "I wish my relationships were different" are some common limiting beliefs. I'm definitely intimately familiar with all of them. The good news is if these limiting beliefs can be caught, and changed to something that propels you, they can always **become empowering.**

"We put a label called 'depression' on something and guess what? We're depressed. The truth is, those terms can be self-fulfilling prophecies."

—Tony Robbins,
Motivational Speaker, Gnarly Tumor Survivor,
Peak Performance Coach

The Most Self-Abusive Belief

People so often develop limiting beliefs about what they're capable of simply because they haven't succeeded at something before. As a result of fear, or past disappointment, they consistently focus on things being "realistic." They develop deep-seated beliefs that connect change or striving for progress to negativity, and stifle their true path to progress and self-fulfillment.

"I don't need to change! Nothing is wrong with me!" was one of my most self-abusive limiting beliefs. This limiting belief can be very dangerous, because anytime we are not willing to even admit that there is a possibility that our short-term beliefs may be inaccurate, we trap ourselves in ideas and life restrictions that could condemn us to long-term fear, anxiety, unhealthy habits, failure, and disappointment. **Nothing has to be wrong for you to want to achieve more, succeed more, and be a better person!** In fact, when you finally recognize how essential growth and progress are in your life, things begin to feel much more "normal" than they ever have before!

One of the biggest challenges in life is how we deal with our personal failures and defeats. After failure, some people begin to believe that their goals, or worse, that *all things,* are pointless, that they're helpless or worthless, or that they will lose anyway. When I was working, studying, adapting, surviving, and strung out on myriad medications, searching for the meaning of life through reckless action, good intentions, and other people, I spent a lot of days wondering, "What's the point?" This destructive mindset is called *learned helplessness*, and it can destroy our ability to act. These thoughts must be caught immediately and replaced with empowering beliefs about what we're truly capable of!

The First Limiting Belief

"Enjoy your own life without comparing it with that of another."
—Marie-Jean-Antoine-Nicolas de Caritat, Marquis de
Condorcet (1743–1794), French Philosopher,
Mathematician, Early Political Science Know-It-All
Whose Ideas Were Said to "Embody the Age
of Enlightenment," Guy Who Really Knew His Shit

At thirteen years old, I definitely began to truly believe some self-destroying things. This is the first year that my childlike wonder completely ceased for what felt like forever. *I believed that other people determined how I felt.* My first year as a teenager, my first year on medication, my first year of surrender, was the first time this thought was solidified for me. I was told by those around me, professionals even, that I was completely helpless to my own thoughts and feelings and mental well-being. I was told that without a pill I wouldn't have a life, be able to get a job, have a relationship, or do well in school, even though I had done all of those things *perfectly fine* before starting lithium. One day, one diagnosis forced me to believe that I was a naturally depressed, naturally unlucky, naturally anxious person. Everyone around me confirmed this. Everyday circumstances confirmed this. And, each and every day, in some way, I confirmed this too.

One of our most common and greatest mistakes is to let other people make judgments about us that in turn compel us to act on those judgments, or to compare ourselves with our fellow humans or our past mistakes. Without faith in yourself, you will lose control of the mental and physical faculties that are required to bring you to your greatest goals and dreams.

COMPARISON

The problem with comparison is that it leads to feelings of inferiority. Inferiority is a distraction from our true purpose. As a woman, you may feel like the woman next to you in class or at work outshines you because she has the best clothes, even if you know that she's an inferior person. The one who suffers may actually possess a greater ability, but she can't recognize it because of limiting beliefs in herself that stem from comparison. This also means, if someone—a friend, a partner, even a stranger—is comparing him- or herself to you, or comparing you to someone else, even if they're comparing you to your former self, *don't entertain them. Walk away.*

I always dated the same type of person. I call them "the Archaeologists" because they're always focused on the past. My boyfriends cared an awful lot about what I said two weeks ago. The girls I dated would constantly bring up who I was *before I even met them.* Sound familiar? People play this game every day and it's one of the most dangerous.

The major key to your better future is walking away from the people who are stuck. Stuck on their personal development, or stuck on yours, stuck on who you were two years ago or yesterday, instead of asking: *Who are you becoming?* This is what separates people who are rich in every way from people who "lead lives of quiet desperation."

In my favorite book as a teenager, *The Perks of Being a Wall-flower,* Stephen Chbosky writes, "We accept the love we think we deserve." This quote struck me particularly hard when I first read the book, and continues to resonate with me even today. Accepting the love we feel we deserve is all about setting new standards for ourselves and the love, home, bank account, friends, career, attitude, and life that we know is already ours. I am here to tell you just what you deserve: **everything you want.**

Jot down five things you feel you deserve right now in the box below. Read them over, and pick the one dearest to your heart. Now, picture your life as though it were already yours.

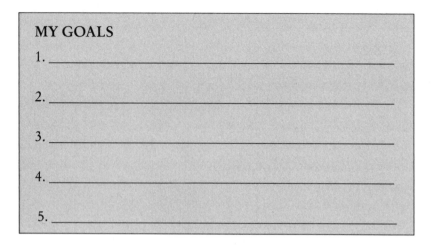

MY GOALS

1. _____

2. _____

3. _____

4. _____

5. _____

This, at first, may be heartbreaking, because your heart desires it and knows you deserve it. But try to swallow your pride for a moment and remember that **you already possess it**. Your book is already written. Your dream house is already built. Your rent is already paid. Your hard work has already paid off. You've made your millions, and there's plenty to go around. All you need is the correct mental adjustment.

Every night before bed for a week, read your favorite goal from your list again and quietly picture yourself—even for a moment— in possession of it. It may be your dream career, your favorite car, the ability to give back to others, or enough money to pay the rent next month. Whatever your heart truly desires, let yourself have it for a few moments.

But, you may ask, won't I be disappointed if I don't get it? Well, that depends on you. **Won't you be disappointed if you never try?** The surest way to not achieving your dreams is to admit to yourself that you don't deserve them. Wake up, you beautiful soul! You deserve it all! Setting higher standards is the way to get there!

The Second Limiting Belief

The second limiting belief I had was that **I was a victim of circumstance**. I was destined to become a drug addict and an alcoholic.

With two drug-addicted parents, the odds of that are 100 percent! "Poor girl, who will never be able to leisurely enjoy alcohol" was the sentiment I heard from family daily. Not semi-regularly. Literally every day it was reinforced to me that I could never touch the stuff, or I'd end up just like my mom.

Today, I can leisurely enjoy a glass of merlot or a pint of beer without going for another, although it's not my preference. If my odds were 100 percent, the Odds Gods miraculously skipped me. But growing up, I heard all around me, "Our genetics are our genetics." "Our past is our past." "We are who we are." "Nobody really, truly changes." And I believed this (drivel!) for a very long time.

Telling yourself things like "I'm a failure" or "I'm going to end up like my father" or "I don't know where I'm going" is the surest way to end up exactly there—like your father, or lost, or whatever place you fear. People have a tendency to receive a diagnosis of depression, and consequently begin to believe that they are naturally depressed. This means that a doctor has told them that they have a "depleted serotonin level," which is often diagnosed as clinical depression, and has in turn prescribed a drug or a series of drugs to increase said "depleted levels."

But what if serotonin is not the issue? What if it is an external factor—maybe that person has begun to eat more sugar and have emotional crashes they aren't used to? Maybe they have a negative mindset from growing up in a negative household. Perhaps the doctor caught them at a bad time. Their spouse may have just passed away. Maybe their mother said something that brought them down that morning.

Let's entertain the fact that serotonin is the issue for a moment. If so, why isn't something like 5-HTP, a serotonin precursor, prescribed? Unlike what I had been prescribed to treat depression, which essentially hands us serotonin chemically and hopes for the best, 5-HTP encourages serotonin levels to develop and be released in us naturally.

Or what about acupuncture, which releases endorphins, dopamine, and serotonin to both stimulate and relax your body as needed?

How about yoga, which has been used for centuries to treat mood swings, depression, and anxiety along with physical and mental illness?

I wasn't given any of those options. The only prescription my doctor had for a "sick mind" was an adult dosage of lithium. In fact, that's all he had been taught to prescribe. Again, I was told that these drugs were vital to my health and necessary for my survival.

I accepted my mood disorder, and I accepted that its answer was lithium without question. The total irony that my grandparents—who had spent years trying to keep me off drugs—were about to start paying to put me on them, was totally lost on me.

I saw this my whole life: the Diagnosis, the Prescription, the Pharmacy, the Trial and Error. Other relatives had played the game for years. Many of us happily do. We're taught—and we desperately want to believe—in a doctor's diagnosis and treatment. We've come to accept this. It's the New Normal. I never thought twice about it for over a decade. With insurance companies, advertisers, pharmaceutical companies, and lobbyists all deep in the game, we're rarely encouraged to search for alternative options to support our wellness, especially options that may be super simple and cost us barely anything at all.

The disruptive truth is, drugs don't teach us anything. As you'll come to read in this book, pharmaceutical drugs are specifically designed to confuse the body as a whole, scrambling extremely important bio-information and essential brain chemicals that control everything from our weight to our moods to our immunity.

But no one ever told me that. The only thing anyone told me was to take lithium. I had to take lithium. If the question of "How Do We Treat Bipolar Disorder in a Thirteen-Year-Old?" had been multiple choice, the options for answers would have been:

A) Lithium
B) Lithium
C) All of the above

Seriously.

Currently, we don't test for depression, manic depression, anxiety, OCD, or any other mental illness the way we do with everything else we medicate for. We don't take a brain scan and say, "Yes! *There* is the anxiety!" or "Here is where your depression starts and here's where it ends." We don't test to see if the drugs we take for mental illness are actually helping our disorders, if we need to switch drugs, or if we really need the drugs. As patients, our diagnosis is an educated guess by our medical professional, at best.

Am I saying there's no such thing as mental illness? Or that drugs are not necessary for cases of mental illness each and every day? Of course not! Psychiatric medication has saved millions of lives. However, there are some alarming statistics about how our country is being medicated: **222 million prescriptions** were filled *in the first three months* of 2014 at Walgreens alone![1] **By the end of 2014, that means Walgreens filled prescriptions for almost three times more drugs than there are people in the country!** *And that's just one pharmacy!*

Unless there is an underlining genetic disorder, the right diet, amount of exercise, and physical activities can give you all the adrenaline, serotonin, and dopamine you need to get through your issues rationally. Especially if your life feels unmanageable, taking a pill does not teach you any new coping mechanisms, does not naturally enhance or organically rewire your brain, and is not meant to guide you on your path to natural wellness. Depending on pharmaceuticals is like putting a Band-Aid on a broken bone. You're NOT helpless to your own mind, and there is a better way.

The Third Limiting Belief

Third, I believed that **illness had no value and it was to be feared.** Fear, too, required medication later on in my life. I saw absolutely no positive lesson in any kind of illness, and fed my diagnoses with more fear. I unconsciously used this fear and these dominating illnesses as excuses for not achieving my deeper goals and dreams, or for limiting myself in some other way.

Once I had the "Manic Depressive" label, I gave it all the power, and all other labels came easily. I was depressed, anxious, worried, pessimistic, sarcastic, crazy, and manic all within the first few months. I was a survivor, a fighter, a threat, or just plain jaded in a matter of a few weeks, all depending on my current thoughts, actions, and behaviors, but it really all came down to one thing: my beliefs. After a while, there was a deep part of me that was scared to live without these labels. What, or who, would I be if I wasn't crazy?

We all have the capacity to create beliefs around events that either make those events empowering or disempowering. Great tragedies, like death, chronic illness, cancer, and abuse, or ones like day-to-day stress, work, or a bad breakup can be recognized as meaningful things with the capacity to shape us positively, if we look at them as such.

Creating these beliefs *must* become a lifestyle. Much like playing music, it is something we must practice over and over and do *consciously* so that it practically plays itself *unconsciously*, on the stage of life, when we're not thinking about it, and we can properly rock out.

To properly rock out in life, we have to unconsciously get in touch with ourselves. It's easier than it looks. Johann Sebastian Bach put it best when he said, "It's easy to play any musical instrument. All you have to do is touch the right key at the right time and the instrument plays itself." Cheeky guy.

If you want to create long-term, conscious, and consistent changes in your behaviors, or your life, your first step is acknowledging and changing the beliefs that are holding you back. Beliefs also interestingly have the capacity to override the impact of drugs on the body.

I read a study recently that truly demonstrates the power of belief: one hundred medical students were asked to test two new drugs. One was described as a sedative, the other, a super-stimulant. Unbeknownst to the med students, the contents of the capsules had been switched: those medical students taking the super-stimulant were actually taking the depressant, and vice versa. Yet, half of the students developed physical reactions that went along with their expectations—*producing the opposite chemical reaction that the drug should have produced in their bodies*! These students—all of whom were studying medicine at the time—were not given placebos; they were given the actual drugs.[2]

Being told that we're dumb often makes us clumsy, being told we're ugly makes us feel less than perfect, being told we're sick often feeds our disease. Our beliefs have the capacity to make us healthy or make us sick in a moment! They've been documented to affect our immune systems, neural pathways, and even our everyday capabilities.

Every single thing that happens to us is valuable. From the most painful to the most pleasurable moments, there's a lesson in them all. We may feel limited in our ability to create a rewarding work experience or a fulfilling relationship. We may feel limited emotionally in our ability to connect lovingly and meaningfully with others, or frustrated with our ability to heal or get well. You might ask yourself constantly, "Why me?" But a better question to ask is, "Why am I on this journey? Why am I blessed with the greater awareness that allows me to be consciously involved and evolving in this healing process?"

Become the Creator

The Bible summed it all up quite eloquently. "Ask and you shall receive." It doesn't say, "Ask desperately and you shall receive," and it doesn't say, "Whine about life and you shall receive." Clarity is power. We have to know what we want before we can begin to ask for it. Once we ask, the power is all ours.

What are your musts in life? Not based on your current conditions or experiences or physical limitations, but what are things you feel that you **must** do before your time on this earth is up? Tony Robbins, the incredible life coach whose scratchy voice was the fly on my wall throughout my tumultuous child-hood, puts it this way: To build an extraordinary life we must have an extraordinary psychology. To do that we must be in an extraordinary state, and to do that we must condition the nervous system to be at its best. We all have the ability to do this, so why doesn't everyone? We all have the ability, but we don't all have the strategy.

The Strategy: Setting New Standards

Once you have a dream only one of two things can happen: it either becomes a reality, or it does not. That gives each and every one of your dreams 50/50 odds and a 100 percent possibility of reality. Isn't that *exciting*?!

I don't believe any of us have dreams that were not given to us for the purpose of accomplishment. Think about your dream right now. Whatever your dream is, however far-fetched it looks, however disappointing your past might have been, know this: your dream is already real. It's possible. Future reality is fertile with possibility. This is one of the greatest universal truths I know.

If you don't make plans and goals of your own, you'll always fall into someone else's plans and goals. This happens to me the moment I slack on myself. I start doing things for other people. I get caught up in other people's emotions. That's because when I slack on myself, I believe, act, behave, and therefore look more vulnerable (because *I am more vulnerable*!) and therefore, I get thrown into other people's lives and plans, instead of focusing on making and accomplishing my own.

When I catch myself, the first thing I check is my philosophy. *What do I believe about myself in the present moment? What standards am I living up to?*

Setting new standards is easy for everyone because it's something we all do every day. We decide when we're going to wake up, what we're going to put in and on our bodies, if and how we're going to move, if we're going to progress, who we're going to talk to, what we're going to do for work, every day. We set standards at practically every moment. We set standards every time we wake up; most of the time they just stay the same.

IT'S EASY

When asked how he became a millionaire by the age of thirty-one, American entrepreneur, author, motivational speaker, and Tony Robbins's mentor Jim Rohn said, *"If you will change, everything will change for you."*

His rags-to-riches story embodies the American Dream, and it was all based on a philosophy he picked up at twenty-five. He even says it was *easy.*

If it's so easy to do, then what's the problem we face? Well, Mr. Rohn also says that the same things that are easy to do, are also easy *not* to do. That's the difference between success and failure, and that's the philosophy that changed Jim's life. If we already do it every day, it's easy. The problem is that most of the time, we're setting our standards *unconsciously.* Once you start to *consciously* set new, higher standards for yourself, setting newer, even *higher* standards becomes easy.

STRATEGIES

The first strategy in setting new standards is to realize that we are the only ones who create our own world and our own reality. You may have heard this before, but in this book, I'm going to help you understand it and apply it to your life. You'll see results instantly if you practice these strategies every day, even if it's for just a few minutes a day.

Our reality is based on our perception and what we allow into our minds. That's where all the shifts happen. Once you make that breakthrough, then it just becomes a game, like life was as a child. You can be anyone you put your mind to be. Life is full of possibility. It's about creating a self-fulfilling ritual: doing a little bit toward your goal and who you want to be each and every day. In doing this, you're creating momentum for yourself with absolute certainty toward who you feel you truly are.

YOUR PASSION

You have to find something that gets you up in the morning. You need to find what you're passionate about, so that you can start your foundation. This passion for life varies for each of us because we all have a different calling. These beliefs are the foundation of developing our self-confidence in our journey of self-discovery.

You may sit in traffic and think, "Nothing is happening to me." Or, you may get frustrated. You may make an important phone call and see it as an opportunity for success. You may pop in a Rosetta Stone and see it as an opportunity for learning, or growth. You can drive around listening to other people's music, or you can cruise around and listen to your own music app creations. Have you ever driven around with someone who is hearing their own music on a stereo system for the first time? It's a magical moment.

Whatever you choose to do in the moment determines what you are taking in. Just like how we metabolize food, in this way we are metabolizing the world around us at every moment: ingesting it in every way. Most of us shape our beliefs about everyday experience based on our past. We carry this into our future, and act on it in our present. These actions then create a result, and that result reinforces the belief we started with, regardless of whether it's positive or negative. The potential to be successful, healthy, nurtured, and loved never changes. It is our ability to exercise the desire to be all of those things that changes. We don't change our potential: that was always with us. **We do change our results, however, by having the certainty that releases our full potential.**

Once I realized that only I created my own feelings, and therefore my own world, *everything* changed. I created a small, meditative ritual for myself to reinforce positive behavior: I started to stop and think before everything I did. Does that mean I painfully paused before the start of every sentence, or second-guessed every move I made? Well, no. As a native New Yorker, and a Virgo, that's *quite* impossible for me *all* the time. However, I did stop drastically. I stopped to appreciate my life, my feelings, and what I was going through. Instead of being completely scared or imprisoned by my fears I faced them in every way I could think of.

TRIGGERS

I used technology to my advantage in my healing process, and I am so grateful we have things like iTunes, the Internet, and tons of free apps, websites, blogs, and media to help us in our journeys and allow us to connect with one another. Things even we Millennials used to dream of doing as a kid (like making my own playlist in five seconds instead of recording it on a tape for five hours then transferring it onto a CD or having our own songs on demand at any time) have been so miraculously helpful.

Music is important to me. I have a very personal and emotional connection to it. In the early days of my recovery, I listened to one song from my past that made me sad, either because it reminded me of something sad from my past, or because it was linked in my memory to a bad experience, followed by either one calming, meditation track or a feel-good, dance-y song that made me happy.

I tried to see the happiness in the sad songs, but on some days I just let them totally absorb me and turn me into a ball of tears. But eventually, I "got over" the songs, I got over the reminders, and I got over the sadness associated with the music too. I owned my moments and I had found a way to do the near-impossible. I controlled my past.

In the process of choosing when and what music I heard, in having a firm grasp on my response to triggers, I had complete control over how I was responding to otherwise upsetting stimuli. Then, when I'd hear a sad song in the grocery store, or someone's car, I wouldn't immediately cringe or have a trigger reaction. This was a very tiny shift, but it was . . . miraculous, and it made me feel awesome.

Life never gives us anything we cannot handle. People who have gone through horrific, traumatic experiences have a willpower, and with the right support and even a small chance, they cannot only survive, they can thrive.

Life's Musts

Make it a priority to list five things that are musts for you right now in your life. For instance, "I must start yoga," "I must write my novel!" "I must start checking my anger!" or "I must sell my paintings!" are all great examples.

This is the only way that we can start to carve out a new path that leads us to the life of our dreams. It is also a great way to evaluate what is important for us, where we're feeling stuck, and what kind of positive change we can begin to work toward.

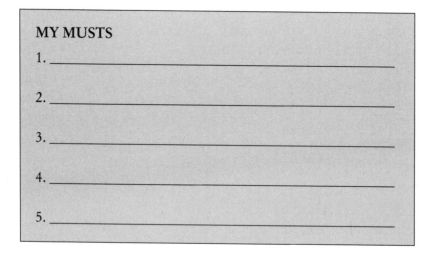

MY MUSTS

1. _____

2. _____

3. _____

4. _____

5. _____

The Fourth Limiting Belief

The fourth limiting belief I had was that I was all alone. No one could ever love or support or comfort me enough. No one would ever understand me. I was never satisfied. I truly believed that without someone else, I was incomplete. I lived in a world dominated by this unhealthy belief. I thought love was in the next boyfriend, the next good grade, or the next promising pill.

I had no idea how I was going to survive without a spouse, so I got engaged at sixteen years old to a boy I had been dating for six months. *He* even proposed! *Those* are the kinds of people I was attracting (boys who propose at sixteen!).

We stayed engaged well into college, but it was possibly one of the most unhealthy relationships I had. Although we loved each other a lot, I couldn't do anything without him. I expected him to solve all of my problems, if not for me, at least *with* me. It never occurred to me that he was not there to do that for me 24/7. That he too was sixteen and maybe had no idea what the hell he was doing either. That boys, in general, have a hard time catching up. I did desperate things for his attention.

I'd regularly do things like drive a three-state distance to see him for our anniversary, then lock myself in the bathroom for hours and wail when I learned he didn't make any plans for us. It didn't actually matter *what* we did together. I always ended up in a ball of tears.

Honestly, I realize now that some people just aren't compatible. It's okay to admit this in your relationship. It's not a failure. It's not a reflection of you or your hard work. It just *is*.

I also see that I wasn't truly alone. He was always there for me at the drop of a hat, in whatever way he was emotionally capable of being. I just always *felt* alone, because I had completely unrealistic expectations of him.

I run into him all the time, to this day. I currently live over three thousand miles away, but whenever I visit home and find myself in New York City I'll be on the subway, in front of Radio City, or in the deli when I'm about to buy kale for my smoothie. I'll look up from my book on the A train, I'll say my blessings to someone who sneezed, or I'll turn to someone next to me in line, and there's his face, slack-jawed, totally as shocked to meet my eyes as I am to see his. We have our WTF moment, and then we move on. We live nowhere near one another, so this has been a constant confirmation to me that clearly, he and I are meant to be in each other's lives. We're just not meant to be married.

Life is certainly not meant to be lived alone, struggling; life is meant to be shared. But this doesn't mean that you *always* need someone around to share it with. *Happily ever after* has all kinds of shapes, names, and faces. Accepting who you are takes a lot of self-reflection, and therefore, a lot of alone time. If you feel like you always need someone around, you will find that this is a way to escape facing your true self.

Other people actually have absolutely no power to make us feel happy—it is our interpretation of them that does. Our beliefs about how special or awesome or cool someone is cloud everything. Once we do start on the path to figuring out our true selves, it's absolutely magical how we attract those who also are on their own journey of self-discovery and reflect what's really valuable to us.

A LIGHTHOUSE

I always longed to be "that girl." You know the one. She walks in the room and all heads turn, because she's just glowing. She's always smiling, optimistic, curious, and everyone else is always talking about how helpful she's been. You can't tell if the glow is coming from the inside or the outside, but you can tell that everyone else sees exactly what you see. It's an inner light.

If you're one of those people who can't help but stop and smell the roses, or can't help but be nice and compliment or aid people, I guarantee you that people will start to stop and smell the roses with you, and you will begin to make friends who compliment and help you right back. I used to think this was rubbish. I'd think, "But I AM nice to people. I do everything for everyone, whenever they ask, and no one appreciates me!"

When I had those thoughts, I wasn't appreciating *myself*. I was bending over backward for others as a way of *escaping* myself. Once you get a true appreciation of life, once you accept good thoughts instead of bad ones, and have a real, true sense of yourself, other people **will** notice. And, trust me, they'll act like they notice.

My favorite Roald Dahl quote really sums it up:

"A person who has good thoughts cannot ever be ugly. You can have a wonky nose and a crooked mouth and a double chin and stick-out teeth, but if you have good thoughts they will shine out of your face like sunbeams and you will always look lovely."

Cultivating a great relationship with myself has been the biggest and most rewarding change of all. Once you've developed an honest relationship with yourself you will notice that you instantly attract other people whose values align with your own, who share in your personal journey, and who walk a parallel path to yours. We are all in this together. Seeking always needs to be directed from within and then shown outward to other people.

Think of your soul, your personality, or your aura as a lighthouse. You are the keeper of the lighthouse. You must remain alert and vigilant, but also shine your luminance constantly. This light is not only for you. It's also a way to let passersby know that even in the stormiest of seas, they have a direction to follow. Others will instantly be grateful for this light; it can save lives.

The Fifth Limiting Belief

The fifth limiting belief I carried through all my life was that **happiness was a lot of work**. Depression had exhausted me, emotionally and physically, so honestly, thinking about doing *anything* was a lot of work.

My tendency during muscle spasms or depressive episodes was to mope around, loaf, watch TV, and hope it passed. I was *waiting* to be happy, like happiness was an elusive true love that hadn't found me yet. I wasn't alone.

Many people spend their lives *waiting* to be happy. I had a bad case of the If-Onlys for years. You may think, "If only I had more money," or "If only I wasn't in pain," or "If only I could lose weight," or "If only (fill in the blank)," *then* I would be happy.

Sometimes, regardless of your hard work or good deeds, life just deals you a bad hand. It's not Karma. It's not because you were a bad person or you deserve it. Shit just happens sometimes. Even for eternal optimists there are some things—chronic illness, death, financial setbacks, or chronic pain, for example—that can lead us down a path of negativity. And being upset, going through things, crying, being angry, and expressing your feelings is *completely healthy*. But people tend to have a cognitive bias toward their failures, and toward negativity. Our brains are more likely to seek out negative information and store it more quickly to memory.

Of course, some of that bias is necessary. Acknowledging and facing our failures often helps us to grow, change, and lead us to better solutions in the future. However, drowning in the negatives and not allowing ourselves a step back is often where even the most motivated of us become the least likely to succeed. During these times, it can be hard to think about anything other than what's wrong. The problem overshadows our whole lives: all of our past struggles turned accomplishments, all the positive reminders that we need to move on, and the perfect people we are get buried in it. We can become so consumed in our own misery that we often overshadow any glimmer of hope that's frantically waving to us.

Having now seen both sides of it, I know for a fact that depression is a lot more work than happiness. A *lot* more. It drains our bodies, confuses us, and gives us an unhealthy perspective not only of others and our life situations, but also of the thing that determines it all: ourselves. We get so wrapped up in either dwelling on the past, or being apprehensive about the future, that we forget to be grateful and focused on the present.

Happiness is not an ever-elusive thing that you need to strive for constantly. It is a new muscle, a fresh hobby, and ultimately, a choice in the moment, every moment, and there are ways to grow it and nurture it, the way you would a plant. Just like plants, we are always reaching for the light, cultivating healthy habits. Making these habits a daily part of our lives is one of the biggest steps to true fulfillment.

Floating on the Positives

"The law of floatation was not discovered by contemplating the sinking of things, but by contemplating the floating of things which floated naturally."

—Thomas Troward (1847–1916),
Mental Science Practitioner, Author, Influencer of the
New Thought Movement and Mystic Christianity

You want the secret to real happiness? *Accept what is happening instead of desiring things to be different.* I call this "Floating on the Positives." When we float on the positives, we finally feel like we are seeing things clearly, because positive, guided thinking is our natural state. We can step back from ourselves without judgment and begin to adjust our attitudes and actions to match the life we know we deserve. We can acknowledge when we mess up, and correct our course without beating ourselves up. Contemplating *what we want* instead of *what we don't want*, thinking about how to make ourselves better, being more loving, caring, and patient, will make it easier for us to manifest what we deserve.

Being honest with ourselves is part of the strategy, but it's not the entire method we use to fight the battle. Being fully present and stopping ourselves from obsessing over things that are out of our control are some of the first steps to ridding ourselves of negative feelings. Here, we begin to find our solutions and fresh perceptions, because we are inviting our mind to be our ally, instead of our enemy.

WHAT YOU CAN'T CHANGE

Here are a few things you can't change: the weather, the past, how other people feel, death (I know, this one especially sucks), and taxes. Everything else is pretty much up to you. The minute you choose to be happy in the moment, over focusing on something happy that is yet to occur or a happy event that happened in the past, you have the true perspective you need to *Be Happy—that ever-elusive thing.*

The reason that this takes work is because everything that you believed up until this present moment is comprised of things that happened in your past. The events that have happened in your life, what you've seen, heard, learned, read, and experienced, are all you had until this present moment to form your perception. It's determined how you've chosen to see things, respond, and behave. The beautiful part is that we can always *change* this. Yes, as mentioned in my experiment with music, we can even change how we view our past.

Just like when we truly learn anything else, happiness is *not fleeting* once you understand it. The very moment that you get your first peaceful and enlightened feeling, and you know you've been putting in the work to get there, you won't want it to leave. Every moment of your life will be happy, even when things are rough. Happiness will be your foundation.

When I first began to change my life, I started to go back to my past experiences during quiet time and meditations and talk to myself. I went back to circumstances in my life that bothered me, and I talked myself through them. I've taken myself back to the darkest hours of my life and relived every gruesome detail, all the while telling myself that I had control, that this was all happening for a reason, that I would survive it, and that it was a life experience designed to make me a better person. What this did was make me notice other things I never noticed about the situation, myself, or my behaviors when I was first in the moment. When I "went back," I took away all the blame for my behaviors—good or bad—and my ability to create new habits improved drastically.

When I think back on them, these periods in my life seem much less daunting now that I am hovering over myself with reassuring words. This makes those memories much less difficult to deal with, because I now feel like I have control over them.

The Grand Scheme

Your life is a beautiful, Grand Scheme. There is no quick fix to a chronic problem. Regardless of what a psychiatrist or MD might tell you, there is no magic pill to relieving mental or chronic illness. Of course sometimes medication is necessary in severe cases. Folks truly need it and I do believe it works and has saved many people's lives. But most pharmaceutical medication is designed to mask the problem, not fix it. Pills or no pills, behavioral tweaks and soul-searching are 100 percent necessary for long-term wellness.

You didn't get ill in a day, *even if you got sick in a day*. Years of mental and physical buildup, of tension, and of unconscious trauma have served to create the illness in our bodies. You won't get better in a day, and frankly, it wouldn't be too emotionally, spiritually, or even physically rewarding if you did.

Finding the silver lining and value in our illness is the key to unlocking our happiness and our personal healing process. It will be an ongoing commitment to work as a team with yourself, family, friends, and healthcare professionals to identify the kinks and knots in the web and to remove them one by one, to free your soul, and thereby free your body of the pain, dysfunction, and pathology that has been created over the years.

Yogananda, the spiritual guru who brought yoga to the West in the 1920s, said, *"Change your thoughts if you wish to change your circumstance. Since you alone are responsible for your thoughts, only you can change them."*

I invite you to come on a journey with me to change your thoughts, and improve your livelihood. If you apply even some of the principles found in this book to your life, you will see instant, positive, drastic, and radical shifts in your everyday experiences and your overall well-being. I am so excited for you! Let's get started.

CHAPTER TWO

BREATH: THE UNIVERSAL HEALER

"One half-minute of revolution of energy around the sensitive spinal cord of man effects subtle progress in his evolution; that half-minute of Kriya equals one year of natural spiritual unfoldment."

—Paramahansa Yogananda (1893–1952),
Task Seeker, Western-Eastern Culture Revolutionary,
Self-Realization Founder, Spiritual Guru to Millions

To be perfectly honest, I used to think that meditation was foolish. I thought I knew it all, even though I had spent years in pain without mindfulness, experienced tons of stress without receiving an ounce of peace, wasted a lot of my time working without any rewards, and suffered from chronic sickness with seemingly no cure. This led me straight to a place of complete breakdown. "Why me?" was the only consistent, daily mantra I ever recited. And it was an incredibly powerful one.

My average workday went the same way regardless of where I worked. There was always the dreaded commute. By my late teens, I *had* to have the best job I could think of at the most prestigious place I could name. This was integral to my self-worth, and it normally involved a long and arduous commute from my hometown on Long Island to New York City. This required a bus or three, a Long Island Rail Road train, two or three subways, and a very long walk. It required getting up sometime between five and six in the morning if I even remotely wanted to look "put together" for work. (I rarely did, anyway. By the time I even got to work, between the weather, the people, and the subway, I was always a mess and barely on time. I can only imagine what 100 percent of my bosses thought of me.)

"Meditation" was a foreign word I associated with people in a different class than I was: Spiritual People. It never occurred to me that applying meditation, breathing exercises, or yoga to my own life would in any way help my moods, ease my pain, or give me a new perspective on my life and situation.

But the truth is, I didn't need to be a "Spiritual Person" — or any kind of person — to change. I was going to find out another hard truth: I had the tools I needed inside me all along. . . .

Fifteen

"You don't need any special reason to feel good — you can just decide to feel good *right now*, simply because you're alive. Simply because you want to."

— Tony Robbins, *Awaken the Giant Within*

I took lithium diligently from ages thirteen to fifteen, and my dosage had been increased from 500 mg to 1,500 mg a day.

Lithium was making me nauseous; just seeing those big pills in the morning could make me gag. The summer before I turned sixteen, I went to a small, selective New York art camp where my medication intake wasn't monitored at all. I simply never showed up to the front desk to get my meds in the morning, and the counselors never said anything to me about it. It was here that I first completely stopped taking my medication.

When I returned home from art camp, I refused to take lithium anymore. I felt better, more alive, colors were vivid and beautiful, my art had never been better, and my mind felt clear. I begged Dr. Brown to let me stay off the lithium. He finally agreed.

Dr. Brown took me off lithium, but he put me on something new. I was switched to a drug called Lamictal, an anticonvulsant drug also used as a mood stabilizer. Lamictal was new to the market at the time and had side effects like blurred vision, clumsiness, skin rash, confusion, muscle pain, irritability, and tics, so I was hesitant. Once again, I was told that this was my best option because without a drug I would not be able to function, even though I had just spent my summer making beautiful art and amazing friends, medication-free.

A few months after starting Lamictal, my thinking became much cloudier. My grades in math, science, and Spanish started slipping dramatically. For the first time in my life, I felt stupid.

I felt less sick on Lamictal than I did on lithium, and the pills were smaller, so I took it, but it never really did anything except make me nauseous if I didn't take it at exactly the same time every day. I became a little less zombie and a little more me, but I still felt empty inside and severely depressed over my family and friend situation, which were both dismal.

I was too weird, too loud, or too manic for anyone to want to be around. I ate lunch by myself in the dance room, watching girls who were prettier than me do things with their shapely bodies I couldn't even hope to do. I spent free periods sneaking in on other people's art classes with my brushes and paints, getting a sheepish and approving grin from the art teacher.

I'd frequently escape my own class with a hall pass, running my fingers nervously over the copy of *The Catcher in the Rye* tucked into my blazer. In an empty bathroom stall for five or ten minutes per class, I'd roll down my knee-high socks, sit on that blazer to avoid getting traces of dust or dirt on my uniform, and read alone. I was desperate for comfort.

It never occurred to me, or anyone else, that this medication switch might be the reason that my moods and some of my grades started slipping.

Sixteen

Lucky for me, I've always been sensitive to caffeine, so coffee was never the jolt I needed in the morning. No, I had pills for that. By sixteen I had been prescribed another drug on top of the Lamictal, for attention deficit hyperactivity disorder (ADHD, now termed a "common behavioral defect" that they say affects roughly 10 percent of children). This new diagnosis surprised everyone, even my grandparents, because I exhibited no symptoms of ADHD aside from my grades changing.

Metadate

"Smart, but not too smart to threaten anything they say."
—Jillian Rose Banks (1988–Present),
American Singer/Songwriter, Timeless Beauty, Badass Bitch

It wasn't clear that the ADHD medication Dr. Brown prescribed—a super-stimulant called Metadate—was interfering with my life until after summer break, when I had to audition for music classes. Side effects of Metadate include loss of appetite, irregular heartbeat, stomach pain, irritability, nervousness, nausea, trouble sleeping, light-headedness, and dry mouth. I had them all.

Not only were my grades not getting any better—I was wired. Photos from that time in my life show huge, dilated pupils. Friends I'd met around that time have told me similar stories:

"I remember the first time I met you! You were bouncing around with a flower painted on the side of your face! You came up to me, gave me a big hug, told me I smelled like an old cat, blessed me in the name of Baby Jesus, and walked away."

Yup. Sounds like me.

I was totally tripping out, I could barely concentrate on finishing a single sentence, but worst of all, I choked at auditions. I'd been on stage since the age of seven—at sixteen, over half my life. The stage was my second home. The Youth Ministry and school theater program where I did shows all my life was just across the street from the house I grew up in with my grandparents.

Just steps away. I could see it from my bedroom window. I mean, how lucky could I get?

I spent every free moment there. I showed up early to every practice, and after just two years in plays, I was getting the leads over people twice my age. At twelve, I landed the lead part of Narrator in our community rendition of *Joseph and the Amazing Technicolor Dreamcoat*. My friends' mothers congratulated me. They had auditioned for the part too.

By thirteen, I had performed at Carnegie Hall. If this caused any contention, I never noticed. I was obsessively dedicated: arriving half an hour early and begging the pianist to go over my parts with me before the rest of the cast or chorus arrived. Soon I learned to play the pieces myself on an old Casio keyboard my mom had won on the radio when I was four. I found a lot of solace, therapy, and healthy escape in musical theater and show business. I could become anyone I wanted, everyone found my voice comforting, and I was *somebody* after the show was over. The only time I ever got praise from even the most judgmental people in my life was when I opened my mouth and sang.

My worst nightmares consisted of not getting the parts I knew I was *meant* to be performing in my final years of high school. At sixteen, on Metadate, I showed up for chorus class to audition for the end-of-the-year show. I had practiced my part so many times I could sing it in my sleep (really). I knew the audition order, because I had asked my teacher at the beginning of the class. I remember waiting for the girl in front of me to finish, anxiously rocking my leg.

As the girl finished and everyone clapped, I looked over at my teacher. She was sitting at the piano with a big smile on her face. She loved hearing me sing and had told me so quite a few times. She said to me once that she was grateful to know me, and knew that I was destined for big things. It meant the world to me at the time, and I still think of it often.

As I walked up to the piano to audition, my hands began to shake. I looked at the music sheet, looked out at the class, and I started to tremble. This had never happened to me before. Not onstage, in front of thousands of people. Not at church in front of everyone I knew I'd see at the grocery store right after Mass. Not in front of people who were more talented than me. Not when I sang for the bishop. Not ever.

First, my hands began to shake uncontrollably. The sheet paper wavered in my hands like there was an earthquake. Then, my knees began to shake! They started trembling like I was going to fall. I held on to the piano, and assured my teacher I was all right. I was still shaking noticeably when she played the intro. And I *missed it*! I just . . . didn't start when I was supposed to start.

"Everything okay?"

"I'm fine."

"Wanna start over?"

"Please."

I could feel people's eyes and hear them whisper. She played it again, and I started on time, but this time, within a few seconds, the trembling started in my throat and my voice cracked. I was visibly shaken. The only other time my voice had ever betrayed me was when I was straining for a note at voice lessons. The teacher kept playing and I kept singing, but I didn't finish. I politely asked to stop, sat down, and let the person after me walk up to the piano. Then I ran to the bathroom to bawl my eyes out.

Heart-to-Heart

Luckily, that teacher was the first one ever to pull me aside after class and ask me what was going on. I had a heart-to-heart with her and my best friend Fiona after class. Fiona told her that I had been on lithium since I was a kid and had just been switched to Lamictal and an ADHD medication.

"ADHD?!" my teacher exclaimed. "You're one of my brightest students! Tara, you don't have *that*!"

At first I argued with her. "But a doctor had told me I had it!" I said.

She told me something along the lines of, "That guy is a quack." And to never apologize for a few bad grades, or let some slipups convince me that something was wrong with me.

After some persuasion, I agreed with her and so did Fiona. The medication was clearly doing more harm than good, *regardless* of whether or not there was something wrong with me.

Results

The next time I had an appointment with Dr. Brown, I told him about my conversation with my chorus teacher, and he listened intently. After a moment, he put his pen down, looked up from his notes, and shriveled his face. He said he was reluctant to take me off of the ADHD medication, specifically *because* we "hadn't seen results" yet!

I had picked up the medication myself more than a few times, and I knew it was costing my grandparents a pretty penny for a bottle, even with insurance. I was a lot sassier with him by then, and I let him know exactly what was on my mind.

"I'm not gonna take the shit anymore, so don't waste their money!" It just came flying out of my mouth like I'd practiced it. This surprised me, because for once I hadn't.

This wasn't the shy thirteen-year-old girl who had first walked into his office three years before with a dirty-laundry diary. This, in his mind, was a defiant teenager with a mental illness, and she was challenging him. I knew adults didn't like to be challenged. I was told by adults all the time that *I had no idea* about life and my childish notions had no place in my education, my health, or my discipline.

Dr. Brown didn't respond to me. He called my grandparents in to talk to them before we concluded our session. I was not invited to this meeting, and instead sat outside the office reading and trying to listen through the wall from my seat, smiling coyly at the secretary. I can guarantee you that this "manic-typical" behavior of defiance was relayed to my grandparents, because I was taken off the Metadate, but my dosage of Lamictal was increased.

Thus my ADHD label was dropped, just like that. But I stayed on Lamictal for the next eight and a half years.

Beliefs

"All I ever want is to be liked," I wrote in my 2003 journal. *"I know that sounds teen angsty and cliché, but it seems like every time I turn my back, someone is figuring out how to hurt me. . . . I think I realized that no one will ever love me the way I need to be loved. And no one ever has."*

These beliefs are echoed in just about everything I wrote for almost a decade after my Lamictal dosage increased. To sit down quietly, to learn myself, and to learn my breath would have sounded like a totally absurd way to help control my pain, mood swings, anxiety, and desperation back then. But I am here to tell you that it's true. Unfortunately, I never earnestly tried it until I was at a complete breaking point in my life.

Even when I was nineteen years old, my journal read, *"I need to meditate more."* But I gave myself excuse after excuse.

Why You Want to Meditate, but Don't (and How to Get Started)

"If you don't run your own life, somebody else will."
—John Atkinson (1844–1931), Irish Politician, British Judge

We all want to meditate because it's really, really good for us, no matter who we are. We spend our whole lives trying to find a universal bandage for things: everything from medication to alcohol, from sex to street drugs, all are ways of finding meaning in our lives and trying to fit all of our ambitions together. What if I told you that the answer lies within you, just a layer below the surface?

You want to meditate because meditation connects us to ourselves. It gives us the tools to deal with all the problems we've been chasing solutions to—forever.

You don't meditate, because you say . . .

". . . I Don't Have the Time."

This was my absolute favorite excuse, and part of that may have been because it made me feel important to be *oh-so-busy* all the time. Another part of it was that I also felt extremely guilty taking time for myself.

For years, starting from a very young age, I had panic attacks daily. It all started when I'd receive an accusation from someone in my family and try to explain myself. All of a sudden my words were interrupted like hiccups: an acute shortness of breath, chest pains, tightness in my ribs and lungs. I left every class in high school and every one in college at least once due to being "set off" at even the slightest idea that I may have disappointed someone, or the idea that I would "have to act." Literally, just the idea of having to take responsibility in a situation I had never handled before left me gasping for air and crying.

Everyday stress is normal, but chronic stress was putting a lot of wear and tear on my body as well as my mind. Being worried, confused, degraded, and deeply buried in various emotional states contributed to my chronic pain, anxiety, panic attacks, illness, and depressive feelings. I was afraid, honestly. I was afraid of living up to my potential, and I was afraid of getting well. In fact, the longer I was sick, the more I convinced myself that something really *was* wrong with me, and the more afraid I became of finding out who I truly was inside.

The most valuable lesson I was ever taught in Catholic school was that *you cannot love another person until you learn to love yourself*. Saying I didn't have the time to meditate was the same thing as saying I didn't have the time to love myself. It was the same as saying that I didn't have the time to fill up my gas tank because I was too busy driving. It was an excuse, plain and simple, and it was running me into the ground. I knew I needed to take care of myself, first and foremost, before I could ever even begin to learn to care about or love anybody else.

The only reason I ever got upset, yelled, couldn't breathe, had a panic attack, got depressed, loafed around, or otherwise hurt myself *was because of the way I was representing situations in my own mind.* If my boss yelled at me, I thought about that experience over and over again. I repeated it to anyone who would listen. I went over ways I could have changed it, torturing myself over what I should have said, or what I would say next time. "Next time" very rarely came; when it did I was always too panicked to execute what I had planned. I thought I *deserved* to wallow, dwell, and feel bad, like that was the solution to all my problems.

Reexperiencing our bad feelings is actually the big thing that is *preventing* us from getting over them. I had never interrupted this pattern of behavior. Instead I clung to unhealthy ways of dealing with stress, like long hours locked in the bathroom, plotting some kind of revenge or dwelling on traumatic past experiences and depressing thoughts. I spent a lot of time crying, or fighting with my feelings, instead of working on ways to soothe myself and make them better. I had all the time in the world; I was just grossly misusing it.

The Same Amount of Time

A mantra is an idea or phrase that we repeat to ourselves to strengthen our goals.

We all have the same amount of time. This was the first mantra that I tackled in my meditations because it really got through to me.

I realized that I had the same amount of time in a day that Benjamin Franklin had, the same amount of time as Gandhi, Jesus, Beyoncé, millionaires, and my mentors. And I had a lot more time than people who had already passed away very early in life, people who had no time left at all. I needed to figure out how to use my time valuably, and for growth. Once I did that, the idea of incorporating meditation into my life came easily to me. It inspired me to finally sit down quietly, focus on my breath, and learn myself. However, that is where I found my next—very common—roadblock . . .

"I Don't Know How"

Uh, okay. *Now what?*

Meditation is not a ride at Disneyland. (Though wouldn't it be amazing if it were? You wait for thirty minutes in line and instead of a children's ride, you walk into a whole room of people in deep meditation with their kids. Where's the Disneyland chill zone? Pretty sure parents *need* this!) The first time I tried to meditate, I didn't like it. I fell asleep, I got distracted, I got bored, and worst of all, I got really discouraged. *"When does this thing start working?"* was basically all I could think for the first week.

Then, I started doing what I do anytime I earnestly want to learn something new: I made a plan. A schedule. A practice. A ritual. I was determined to make it work. Determination is what separates wanting to do something from actually going out and doing it.

When I was a kid I "meditated" all the time to get through my problems. I lost myself for hours alone, drawing, writing, or making music. Before video games, five hundred TV channels, a computer in my room, or a cell phone in my hand, I had known how to get in touch with myself and calm down, at least a little bit. If I had managed to do it as a little kid with a few Tony Robbins tapes and an hour of *Oprah* five days a week, I could definitely handle it with all the resources I had as an adult.

I didn't have many goals or plans when I first began to meditate, other than to actually get that "blank slate" in my mind that everyone was talking about, and to do so on a schedule.

I made a plan that I could stick to: every day after work for at least one hour I would turn off every electronic device in my house, make my bed, light a candle, sit up quietly, and close my eyes.

I let this take me wherever it wanted to at first. I wrestled all sorts of ideas I couldn't let go of. The more I tried *not* to picture something, the more vividly it showed up. The more I tried to clean the slate of my mind, the more all my problems surfaced.

This is normal. It will even happen deep into your practice if you, for whatever reason, stop meditating. The blank slate does not just "show up." We have a million problems, from bills to self-image, from relationships to work schedules, that threaten our peace of mind.

The blank slate came when I made it something I could relate to. I turned it into a black, dark stage, like the ones I had performed on as a child, or had seen at a Broadway show. Then, I turned my attention to it quietly, the way I would if I were patiently waiting for a show to start. I left myself alone in the audience, and just watched. If my problems or the people I was having issues with appeared on the stage, I kept watching until some shadowy figure came and dragged them off. I even pictured this as a silly dance number, to make my problems seem even less daunting.

Later, I replaced those shadowy figures with janitors, coming to sweep my problems away. Then, I pictured them as angels, swooping in to intervene with any roadblock that threatened my amazing livelihood.

I found that it helps a lot of people to think of this as a blank screen, like one at a movie theater.

While staring at this "screen," I focused on my breath. Just breathing in and out at first let me acknowledge where all those panic attacks were coming from: my breath was unsteady, uneven, and it shook with every inhale. Every exhale was practically a gasp. And this was my normal, relaxed breathing! I couldn't believe it! I had been breathing this way unconsciously for years!

Not only that, I had already learned more about my body and my health in the first few seconds of earnestly practicing meditation than I had learned my whole life! After the initial shock wore off, this gave me my first goal.

The Identification Meditation

Sit up straight in your chair with your feet firmly planted on the ground.

Breathe In and feel areas in your life where your emotional discomfort may be manifesting physically. Take a moment to acknowledge those areas, and picture them hugged by light.

Breathe Out: I release all dis-ease.

Breathe In: I am light.

Breathe Out: I release all dis-ease.

Breathe In: I am light.

Continue to picture your unease, emotional distress, or physical discomfort bathed in light with each inhale. Release this dis-ease with each exhale. Practice this for at least seven breaths.

When you are ready, open your eyes and greet your day.

The First Goal

There is no wrong way to get well. Whatever works for you, very fortunately, works for you. The Western idea that medicine must be working on a mass scale and help everybody the same way has been harmful for our culture. At the very least, it has been harmful for *me*.

My first goal was to remind myself that I am allowed to get well in whatever fashion I choose, and to bring people into my life that support those things, rather than to consistently battle people, my body, my environment, my time, my learning curve, my energy level, and my own mind.

The first goal is to give ourselves space to learn. Many of us are frightened at the idea of learning who we really are. Or, we're scared of ideas like alternative treatments, herbal remedies, positive thought practices, or forging our own paths to self-improvement—ideas outside our normal perception of wellness.

That's because wellness is generally learned in our society. It's cultural. We learn what it means through our families, our medical practitioners, and the media. Western medicine, for instance, relies heavily on drugs and treatment instead of preventive care and natural remedies. "Wellness" is seen as a lifestyle, instead of an essential practice. We rarely incorporate wellness into our moment-to-moment experiences.

I invite you to explore how you react, how you speak, and what you're putting into your body for fuel. I invite you to listen to what tones you use, what you've loved about your life, what things you feel stuck on, or whatever questions might serve you.

There is no "wrong" way to meditate, but perhaps meditation wasn't giving you the benefits you expected. That's why most people stop. There aren't really any immediately visible benefits if you are getting frustrated in the process, or worse, if you stop completely. Stopping completely is the surest way to not see any results at all! The first goal is to throw all your previous notions about meditations and affirmations completely out the window, and start focusing **on you**. *What does wellness mean to you? What are you lacking right now that you would like to have?*

The idea is that, along with whatever therapy you choose, genuinely spending your time relaxing your body and mind will help you feel better and shift your focus onto how to better heal yourself in the future. The idea that you create your own wellness is very *empowering*.

"It Hurts"

Many people who experience chronic illness feel that this method of wellness is not for them because it hurts them to sit or stay still for long periods of time. I, too, experienced physical pain. By the time I earnestly started my meditation practices at twenty-four years old, the list of medications I was on had grown substantially. I was still on Lamictal, but most of the medication was for pain from rheumatoid arthritis, fibromyalgia, anxiety, chronic muscle spasms, and the sharp, shooting pain I experienced from my scoliosis. The curve in my spine had become so severe that the muscles on my right side had been pushed under my shoulder blade from the force of my spine, and I was plagued daily by unceasing pain that no amount of narcotic or muscle relaxer or painkiller had ever taken away.

I spent so much time in pain, I could no longer remember what life felt like without it. I brought this pain into every other area of my life—relationships most of all. I took it out on myself and other people all the time.

Own It

The first time I tried to meditate in lotus position, it *did* hurt. This is what scares us at first, because we think, "How can I possibly be sorting my life out if I feel pain when I'm trying to relax?" A valid question.

What I quickly learned was that the pain was going to be there *regardless* of what I was trying to do. It's been there all along, *even if it hasn't yet become chronic.* Chronic illness is underlying. We can mask it, ignore it, treat it, talk about it, but it's always either getting better or worse.

Our bodies should be in perfect balance and alignment all the time because *they are biased toward health and recovery.* So if you experience pain during your meditation process, this now gives you *all the more reason to meditate.* For now, at least, you are working toward getting control back.

I say, do the counterintuitive thing: focus on it. Focus on where it came from and what it means. "Play" with it. If it's a muscle, tighten and relax it. If you can't, work on getting to the point where you can. If you're experiencing nausea, let yourself feel nauseous, but actively try to find out where the nausea's coming from. It was in doing this one night that I realized some of my chronic nausea stemmed from my back being misaligned!

And lotus position? Well, it is now my absolute favorite way to meditate. You must work *through the pain* and then immediately go back to your practice. The point is to *own* it, instead of feeling like your body owns *you*.

Release

Meditation is not about knowing exactly *how* you need to change: it's about learning *why* you need to constantly change and grow. I've waited days to see that "blank slate" clearly; I've played around with my muscles, especially on days where I felt that I could not take the agonizing, throbbing pain in them any longer.

Whenever I got to my breaking point, I focused on releasing my pain, by using daily practices, such as picturing it melting away. Soon, I started doing my meditations in a warm bath, so that I could focus on the warmth outside of my body and create a warmth within that I could easily access to help ease my pain, and one that I could conjure up when there wasn't a bath available to me (when I'm traveling, for example).

After a week or two of these kinds of meditation practices plus morning dancing and stretches, I had my first breakthrough. I didn't reach for the muscle relaxers or the pain medication anymore when I was hurting, because I wasn't hurting even remotely the same way. Most of the sharp, shooting pains turned to dull, achy ones. It had gone down in scale from a ten to maybe an eight during the first week alone. When I was hurting, I took myself to my meditative state and I relaxed, focusing my energy away from the pain, or sometimes picturing an army attacking and dismantling it. This helped me more often than not.

On the off chance that it didn't help me, it was because I didn't believe in what I was doing. Anytime I reverted back to thoughts like, "This can't possibly work," those thoughts manifested, and my practice went accordingly.

Instead of results for two days, my results would be down to one day. I'd find more negative or nagging thoughts popping up during my quiet time or daily life. I knew there was a direct correlation between the daily time I was taking to relax and sort out my issues, and my ability to have a calm, relaxed attitude. And that made a lot of sense to me.

Negative thoughts are inevitable when pain is extreme, but we must resist them. This kind of negativity about our pain clouds our minds, but I reminded myself to believe in the power I had within me. I knew I had gotten myself into this mess, and I knew only I could get myself out of it.

Getting Out of It

It's easy to overcomplicate this, but the truth remains—if you're in pain, do one small thing during quiet time, or meditation time, each day to focus on this pain in a positive way: figure out how to control it so that you can then release it. Even if this seems impossible, even if you've been told your problems are permanent or genetic, even if you think that the pain has complete control over you, remember that it doesn't. Your pain—mental, emotional, physical, or spiritual—was co-created with the connection between your mind and your body, and it can be undone.

Jesus didn't heal people with his hands. He healed them through their own beliefs. That is why he'd ask his followers, "Do you believe in me?" before he healed them. He acknowledged that the sick feel helpless and hopeless, and must therefore give themselves over to another idea of power. It was belief that healed the poor, sick, blind, and dying. Not another person.

Even though I was now super psyched at having control of this immense power to heal myself, it led me to another roadblock that's very common in novice yogis . . .

"It's Boring!"

Well, sure it's boring—depending on your definition of boring. Meditation is now one of the most exciting things I do with my days, but if you're used to the overstimulated life we're all subjected to daily, it's not going to bring you that same stimulation, because meditation is not about that. It's not an action-packed movie and it's not Ryan Gosling or Olivia Wilde making googly eyes at you (don't you kinda wish it was, though?).

Meditation is all about learning ourselves.

And during the process, we often learn things about ourselves we had no idea were true! Just as I learned that I had been breathing in a panicked way for years, with enough time spent focusing on yourself, you'll learn how your own unconscious daily habits have built up dis-ease in your body. Meditation often brings new insights that only quiet time affords us.

If meditation seems boring, if it's not working, or if it's putting you to sleep, let it—but don't give up. You may, in fact, be avoiding yourself, or overlooking the ways in which it *is* actually helping! Ironically, I complained of insomnia, and then I'd complain when I'd fall asleep during meditation! It wasn't until months later that I realized my body was *doing exactly what I needed.* There are valuable lessons in every single thing we perceive as failure.

Practice

Meditation encouraged me to unplug my TV and never look back. These kinds of on-demand distractions no longer appealed to me. In fact, turning on the television started to give me a lot of anxiety! I realized that TV had mostly depressed me. I was ready to replace sitting in front of it with a new practice.

War and Peace wasn't the first book you picked up when you first learned to read, I bet you couldn't play Beethoven when you first laid your hands on a piano, and I assume you didn't learn to drive on a racetrack either. Meditation, like everything else, is something that gets easier with earnest practice. We call meditation a "practice" for that very reason: you are practicing it each and every time you do it.

Meditation is so exciting because it is all the realms, all the possibilities, and all the pain-free, positive circumstances that could ever happen to you. It is precisely what you focus on.

Meditation gets easier each and every time you do it. Just like working a new muscle, you are exercising your brain and teaching it how to relax and start to work *for you*. I have a vast imagination, so picturing a better life has always been, and will be, easy for me. As easy as this part was, practicing meditation earnestly and having to convince myself over and over again that what I was doing was meaningful brought me to my final, and most destructive, roadblock . . .

"That's Hippie Shit and It Doesn't Apply to Me!"

Whether it was my schooling or society putting saints above all the rest of us "born with sin," whether I thought I didn't deserve it, or whether I just wasn't ready to accept responsibility for my own feelings, I shared the thoughts many of us have about meditation: that it's "not for us." I was the most skeptical, learned, holier-than-thou hardass scientist there was, touting my thick Darwin books everywhere I went and preaching Godlessness to anyone at the bar who would listen. I thought my combination of Catholic indoctrination and hard-hitting of the bio books during college made me some kind of expert on dealing with myself. Leave the spirituality on the side, please. And I'll take the check!

Wrong, sister. So, *so* wrong.

Many people think that meditation is only for certain people because it conjures up ideas of spirituality that many folks have never believed in, don't identify with, or have just plain abandoned. So many of us hold ourselves back by believing that our pain, our problems, our life situations, our past are far better, more extreme, or very different than what everyone else is going through, and that they can't possibly be fixed by *thinking about them.*

I used to think that my life was much harder than the lives everyone else led. This was something I actually took pride in. I took solace in my hurt. I thought no one else could ever understand me, and even though it was a lonely life, it made me special. I thought that no one could possibly feel what I felt based on what I had seen, heard, and experienced in my life.

"Making it" in my hometown of New York City, or any city, county, or small town, does require a certain kind of mentality. We start to think that spending quiet alone time is impossible, or can't possibly have a positive impact on our lives, and that we're doomed to this kind of life, pain, or persistent sadness forever. It's easy to feel like there's not enough time, not enough resources, not enough money, and everyone you've ever met has shortchanged you. This is the most harmful place to be in. It is also one of the easiest mentalities to succumb to, especially when we're depressed or experiencing chronic pain.

Jim Rohn's words echo mine here: "What's easy to do is also easy NOT to do." That's why Mr. Rohn got rich in just six years— admittedly he'd "messed up" by the age of twenty-five, but became a millionaire at the age of thirty-one—while the economy, the government, circumstances, unions, and the people around him all stayed the same. However, amid it all, *he changed*, and he taught a very valuable lesson through it: if you will change, everything will change for you.

Ending the Struggle

Wanting to have a handle on your life comes back to one big idea: ending the struggle. The struggle for a job, a promotion, a degree, a marriage, a healthy relationship, or a supportive community ends only when we really want it to. When we really want the struggle to end. When we truly want all the things in our life that we are unhappy with to change.

If you change, nothing around you *has to* change. You don't have to change your circumstances, you don't have to change your income, you don't have to change your dreams, you don't have to change anyone else—that struggle is *over. You alone* need to change in order for everything to change *for you.*

So, why didn't anyone around Mr. Rohn become a millionaire by thirty-one? They *stayed the same.* If you stay the same, your circumstances, your bank account, your company, your clique, your support group will all also stay the same. I lived like this for most of my life because I did not believe that any of my circumstances were up to me to solve. Every single day that I woke up looked just like the day before it. It was a boring, confined, depressing life, and it's unfortunately the norm.

If you want the next two years to look different than the last two years, if you want them to look the way you've always deserved, keep trying to better your life, your income, your fortune, your dreams, and your opportunities.

This is easy. Easy, meaning *something we can do.* I don't know anyone who cannot focus on his or her breath. I don't know anyone who can't picture his or her life better than where it is right now.

Regardless of how successful or satisfied we are, there is always plenty of room for growth and more abundance. You can always love more, appreciate more, and live more fully. You can always want to become more. You do not have to feel guilty about wanting this; it's natural and nurturing and satisfying. Plants seek this every day—that is why a rose is always reaching toward the sunlight.

It doesn't matter what you believe in spiritually; if you come into contact with God, Spirit, or a higher power during your meditations, consider yourself **very** lucky. This is what millions of swamis, monks, nuns, priests, and devotees of all kinds dedicate their lives to and pray for daily. It's an awakening, beautiful experience, but it's not quite the point (unless that's what you're seeking).

The Point of Meditation

I would have done anything to relieve the pain I was experiencing when I first started meditating. I had worn a back brace for three years, gone to ten years of physical therapy, had a dozen X-rays done, been on every medication in the book, and was withdrawing from over a dozen different prescription medications when I first dedicated my meditation sessions to feeling physically well.

A month before I first set my butt on a meditation pillow, I was chewing on prescribed fentanyl patches. These are mostly for cancer patients who suffer from immense pain and are supposed to be placed on a painful area, delivering a fast-acting narcotic straight to the spot. I didn't have cancer, but my pain area was all over my body and sunk into my bones, and these patches didn't do *anything* for me that way. I had to chew on them (a method that has contributed to countless overdoses and one I would never recommend!) to feel anything, and I was always vomiting violently afterward. I didn't even care.

Two weeks after I began my meditations, I didn't reach for a single thing to cure me from my pain. I had learned how to relax. A month's worth of fentanyl patches were part of the medication I gave up completely less than eight weeks after I began earnest daily meditation.

I learned a really valuable lesson that first month of meditation. The empty feeling that I had wasn't going to be satisfied by food, success, education, sex, money, acceptance, relationships, or even love. I had experienced these things over and over again and felt deeply, terribly disappointed. The deeper hunger I had was revealed only when I was willing to relax and learn myself, and it came down to a choice. It was the choice between feeling torn and conflicted, and feeling whole and an immense sense of oneness with my circumstances and environment. This is a choice and a question none of us should be willing to postpone: we've been asking it since the day we forgot what we are really doing here.

"I Don't Know Why I'm Here!"

The last roadblock I faced in my meditation practice was the feeling that I had no idea what the hell I was doing, or why. Especially when it really started to work, and I felt awesome, I had the hardest time remembering *why* I was doing it to begin with. I started to think I could stop meditating *because* I finally felt really good. Luckily, we're all here for the same reason, so regardless of where you're at in life, you've come to the right place for your answer.

It doesn't matter what kind of work you do, you're here to be a light. You're here to be a Creator—that is your greatest purpose. Being a Creator enables you to fulfill your greatest destiny—that is to help others.

The Self-Love Meditation

Sit up straight in your chair with your feet firmly planted on the ground.

Wipe your mind clean and start over. Picture yourself as the most peaceful, calm, best person you can envision.

Breathe Out: I release doubt.

Breathe In: I am love.

Breathe Out: I release doubt.

Breathe In: I am love.

Continue to picture yourself as the most calm, peaceful person you know. Picture yourself surrounded by light, and giving light to all you touch. Practice this vision for at least seven breaths.

When you are ready, open your eyes and greet your day.

You can be anyone or anything you make up your mind to be. Happy, successful, loved, and admired are just a few of them!

Jobs

I've had all kinds of jobs. By the time I started meditating, I had been an account executive, a model, a waitress, a janitor, an administrative assistant, a session vocalist, a scientist, a pizza place phone operator, an actress, a bartender, a hostess, a musician, a physical therapy assistant, an undercover journalist, a grocery bagger, a coat-check attendant, and a lab analyst, among other things. I had worked everywhere from the bathrooms at my local pool changing tampon boxes and scrubbing shower drains to the labs at Weill Cornell Medical Center in New York City.

At the point where I started considering meditation, I was the sole lab technician for an environmental laboratory. After a year at that job, I had started messing up just about everything. I handed specimens over to my supervisor one day, and not five minutes later he called me into his office.

"What's this?" he asked.

"What do you mean?" I was honestly baffled. I had spent the last six hours prepping these samples for him to analyze. They were perfect.

"Are you kidding me?" He slid a petri dish my way. "What *IS* this? Tell me where this corresponds in your logbook. I am asking you what this says."

I looked down at it, and on the petri dishes there was nothing but scribble. One dish after the other had what looked like a combination of kindergarten scrawl and hieroglyphs instead of the label numbers.

I was startled. I couldn't possibly have spent the last six hours labeling all the petri dishes in scribble, could I? There was no way to correspond *any* of the samples to their original specimens.

I could barely get a word out. Instead, I blamed everything and everyone around me. I took a bottle out of my purse that I had just filled the day before. It was a new prescription provided after a doctor was convinced that I had fibromyalgia on top of the other diagnoses—anxiety, depression, bipolar disorder, juvenile rheumatoid arthritis, chronic fatigue syndrome, anemia, hormone imbalance, precancerous cells found in my uterus—that I was facing daily. I hadn't even had the time to look up what the medicine was, or what it did, I told my boss. I had just added it to the regimen. Clearly it had been fucking me up.

I don't think I said I was sorry one time.

I complained, I cried, and I watched my boss's face turn from anger to concern. Luckily, I didn't get fired that day, and I did have to do all the work again, but I *still* didn't learn my lesson. I continued almost all the medicine I was on, I continued to fuck up at work, I continued making excuses, and I continued to cry and complain every time I was confronted with my mistakes.

The Almost Breakthrough

A week after the hieroglyphic petri dish mess-up, I came home from a long day at work and my apartment was covered in ants. They were crawling up my walls, out of the sink, trailing into the garbage can. For almost three hours, I was totally unfazed. I had better things to worry about: my favorite show was on and my boyfriend and I were fighting. I was frantically texting him, filled with empty rage. I popped another pill. It was easy to ignore absolutely everything.

Then, I saw the ants crawling into my dog Raelie's food bowl. I had adopted Raelie on my twenty-third birthday. She was the runt of the litter, the ninth of nine puppies. When I adopted her, she was seven weeks old, had an eye infection and two types of ear infections, was bloated, and could barely walk. Although I raised her as I would my own child, gave up whatever social life I had to care for her, and based everything I did and everywhere I lived on her presence in my life, it had never felt like I'd given *her* the life she deserved. She's half pit bull, and she's been judged from day one.

When she was small enough to carry in my arms around the grocery store, a woman came up to me in the fruit aisle saying that seeing Raelie gave her PTSD (post-traumatic stress disorder). She told me that she had lost a finger to a pit bull ten years ago. She showed me her injury, holding half a finger an inch from my nose, and told me that my dog was a killer, and it was only a matter of time before I realized it. Eight-week-old Raelie slept quietly in my arms, her puppy tummy resting in my right hand, her snout nuzzled and snoring into my neck. I was horrified, but it wouldn't be the first or last time I would hear this kind of thing from strangers.

It felt like we were always sneaking around, never accepted, shade cast over us everywhere we walked or tried to play. Raelie was, and continues to be, the closest thing I've ever had to a daughter. She's not your average dog. Raelie is intuitive. She knows I'm sick before *I* know I'm sick. She has saved my life, provided emotional and physical support, cuddled me every time I needed it, licked my tears away every time I've been upset, lain with me for days when I was sick, and she continues to show me adventure is possible in life.

Waking Up

After seeing ants crawl into Raelie's food bowl, I officially woke up. I loved her more than anything in the whole world, and I finally realized that this could have been happening for days and I wouldn't have even noticed. I couldn't even remember the last time I had fed myself something substantial. I finally saw the terrible pattern of behaviors that had brought me to where I was. I saw how much I relied on pills and other people for my happiness and self-worth. Not only did the pills not help me, they were a distraction. They constantly led me to more pills, more problems, more therapy, and more health concerns.

I realized that my lifestyle was affecting not just me, but many, *many* things that I loved. I was tired of hurting them, and I was really, really sick and tired of being sick and tired.

Thinking that I was a slave to a pill and that I was beyond help were some of the most destructive thoughts that I had. Based upon my new belief that I created my own mentality, that I deserved to get well, and that pills were not my answer, I finally decided to quit all the medication I was on cold turkey. I was finally about to quit more than a dozen pills that I had been on since I was a kid, at twenty-four years old and around 103 pounds.

This is a method that I do not recommend to anybody, because—as you will come to see—I risked my own life many times doing things the cold-turkey way, especially in moments when I really did not want to die. I should have slowly wound down, consulted a doctor to finally get a good, long-term plan for my health, or at least made a treatment plan for myself before I started. But I didn't.

Luckily, I came out alive. And this book is my honest account of what I *did* do. Meditation was the first tool I utilized that really changed my mentality, allowed me to connect with myself, and helped me get where I had been trying to go for years.

I don't want anyone to reach their breaking points before starting their journey, so I encourage you to start now, before you "have to" start. Maybe you *are* at a place where you feel like you have to start. Maybe you've also exhausted all your resources and are at your wit's end. Meditation is a valuable tool that can bring you the life you deserve even if you are on top of the world. It is especially valuable when you are overwhelmed, lost, ill, sick, or confused about your next step.

The Connection Meditation

Sit up straight in your chair with your feet firmly planted on the ground.

Wipe your mind clean and start over. Place one hand on your heart and one hand on your abdomen.

Breathe In and feel where your air flows in your body. Is it just in your lungs, or does it fill your stomach, your abdomen, or other parts of your body?

Breathe Out: I am connected.

Breathe In and focus on smoothing your breath.

Breathe Out: I am connected.

Continue to focus on your breath. Anytime your mind wanders, bring your attention back to your breath.

When you are ready, open your eyes with a smile and greet your day.

CHAPTER THREE

THE BREAKTHROUGH

"The man who has not found Brahman is like the fish who has not found water."

—Ancient Indian Proverb

When I first decided to come off all my prescription medications, I had absolutely no idea what I was in for. There is (literally) no guidebook out there for pharmaceutical withdrawal.

By the age of twenty-two, I was exhausted, defeated, guilty, confused, and had half a dozen diagnoses. I had done my best at three colleges.

I got into Bennington at the age of seventeen, which was both a dream and a nightmare for my grandparents. It was a 550-acre campus in the middle of Vermont. Rolling hills, gorgeous landscape, progressive professors, no tests, and no grades. I'd attend small classes, receive mentors, and get evaluations at the end of term about my progress. It was great for a teenager with a lot of callings who needed just a little push and direction.

Matching Bennington's 550-acre campus were its carefully selected five hundred students—making up the elite of young and forward-thinking artists, writers, and musicians. Most students were the children of celebrities or executives, but some—like myself and a handful of good friends I made there—were just Hardworking Creatives. Both its undergrad and graduate programs thrived in progressive thought and boasted various celebrity alum, from Betty Ford to Bret Easton Ellis.

However, there was Bennington's $45,000-a-year price tag. This was *more than my family earned* in a year. And that was just for tuition. Never mind room, board, meal plans, books . . .

I somehow achieved enough in scholarships and financial aid to make it affordable for my grandparents, but it was a stress game I played with myself every year. *If only I knew if I was going to be able to afford to go back to school . . .*

By the age of twenty-two, I had worked myself to the bone at a ton of completely different jobs I hated and I felt trapped by a different university and the daunting New York City lifestyle. "Debt" was the *only* four-letter word in my life, and relationship trouble haunted me everywhere I went. Physically, I was plagued by frequent headaches, blackouts, anxiety attacks, and unexplainable, excruciating pain diagnosed as juvenile rheumatoid arthritis and fibromyalgia. The idea of ever graduating from college with a degree I was proud of or getting a good job in a field I loved was a pipe dream. It was taking everything I had—and I didn't have very much left.

"Most of the things worth doing in the world were declared impossible before they were done."
—Louis Brandeis (1856–1941), American Supreme Court Justice, Outspoken Lawyer, Harvard Graduate at Twenty Years Old

Relationships

By my early twenties, I found myself in a very abusive relationship with someone who hurt me every way I could think of—first physically, and then emotionally and psychologically, for over *three years*. This certainly wasn't my first rodeo in a bad relationship. In fact, most of them had gone pretty horribly. In many of my other relationships, I had been okay with my breakups. Most of my exes and I were still friends after we had ended things, before this new, toxic relationship began.

My new boyfriend had forced me to cut out just about everyone who was "a threat" to him from my life. Because he was in his early twenties and I was his first girlfriend, everyone was a threat. I was highly encouraged to end all of my friendships. I did.

In the past, I had often been able to shrug off ending a relationship by justifying to myself that we clearly didn't belong together. This new relationship was different: I was dependent and became extremely afraid to leave. Even though I knew that this was the most toxic, unhealthy relationship I had ever been in, I had absolutely no desire to end it. It was my manifestation of a cry for help.

In the first month of our relationship, during our first innocent fight, my boyfriend pinned me to the bed. He was in a terrible rage, screaming at me. He spit in my face and punched me. Then, he pinned me in between the bed and the wall and started choking me. It wasn't until I bit him so hard on the shoulder that I made him bleed that he hesitated. It wasn't until I started screaming at the top of my lungs for help in his small Astoria apartment, hoping that someone would hear me, that he "woke up," and literally ran out the door in fear. I cursed after him, spitting, and a sober part of me realized that *my boyfriend had just tried to kill me.*

Safety

Independent, wild, free-spirited, confident native New Yorker Tara was letting some asshole with a control complex run her life. And she was doing it happily! This Tara was done with responsibility, she was over facing herself, and she was really afraid to realize her true potential.

Even though I got a restraining order against this guy after that incident, it didn't stop me from seeing him, relying on him, or giving into irrational decisions involving him for *three more years*! We even showed up to our restraint hearing together, like a bad Lifetime movie. He did everything he could to exert power over me, from sabotaging my auditions, to spreading rumors about me, to hacking into my email, to guilt trips and more acts of physical violence. Even when I showed his friends police photographs of his fingerprints around my neck. Even when he called the cops *on me*, telling them *I had assaulted him* and I spent a *few hours locked in a holding cell in jail*. Even after I filed my own police report, no one seemed to have any sympathy for me.

This was happening because I had absolutely no sympathy for myself. I would still see him, go out with him, and go out of my way for him, despite the very real fact that this person *actually tried to kill me*, had held me back from accomplishing all of my dreams, and turned me into a completely different person than who I was happy being.

This toxic relationship was something that I clung to for safety. I did not know who I was without this person, and felt like every negative word, every horrific action, and every scary night was somehow a crazy validation that I was loved, because someone cared enough to be mad at me.

A College Dropout with a Shitty Job

At twenty-three years old, I was watching each and every one of my dreams go down the drain day by day. Every day I took one step forward and four steps back. I was always a day older and two days farther away from my goals.

I was on so many pills I couldn't even count them or remember what they all did. I didn't know what worked and what didn't work. I spent half my days in a zombie-like haze and the other half sleeping, complaining, or on hold with or sitting in front of a doctor. Every time I expressed distaste for life with a doctor, I went home with more pills.

I turned twenty-four years old on the first of September. I commiserated with many of my friends, including Fiona and our best friend Grey, about being "a college dropout with a shitty job," but it didn't really matter; many of my friends who *had* graduated with great degrees couldn't find jobs either. People were going to graduate school just to avoid being unemployed. It often felt like we were always competing over who was the most miserable.

The United States represents 5 percent of the world's population, but we consume 50 percent of the world's pharmaceuticals. My friends and I traded prescription drugs with no guilt. After all, these pills had been prescribed to help us! We all felt the same, and those drugs had been given to us for our *feelings.* It was not uncommon to trade some Xanax for some weed, or Valium between my friends. I had seen it since high school.

Understanding

On January 3, Fiona called me. She was sobbing.

"It's Grey . . ." she said, between tears. "I can't . . ."

Grey was one of my best friends, and also an ex-girlfriend of sorts. Grey and I had a great friendship as well as a brief romantic relationship. She was a wonderful girl from my hometown whom I not only loved with all my heart, but also admired greatly and looked up to. She had been in my life for almost a decade. Grey was a chemical engineering major who worked at Cornell on Alzheimer's research during the summer months, constructed physics projects for fun, and was always down for a late-night drive. She was a beautiful, intelligent, wise-beyond-her-years young woman I had spent many incredible moments with.

The only contention we ever had was that Grey never wanted to tell anyone that she was with me. Specifically, that she was with a girl. She was terrified of her family finding out. This was a huge problem for me at the time, and we ended up deciding to remain friends. Last I heard, she had a boyfriend.

"She did it," Fiona sobbed. "She fucking did it."

Grey had come home from her apartment in Rhode Island, walked up to her childhood attic, put her father's gun to her head, and pulled the trigger. It happened just a few blocks from where I grew up. I couldn't breathe.

This violent suicide was not only life-shattering to me, it was life-awakening. The next week of my life was a complete haze. Fiona and I did everything we could to soothe Grey's family and plan her wake and funeral. I had no idea how I was ever going to sleep, eat, or look anyone in the face ever again. I was devastated.

The day before Grey's wake, Fiona texted me:

It's going to be an open casket. I'm just warning you, it said.

I texted back, *How?!*

Fi responded, *I have no idea. I just found out.*

We could never imagine someone who committed suicide this way ever wanting to have an open casket at their funeral, but we went through with it anyway.

And there she was. I stared at her beautiful face and touched her cold hands as they lay on her favorite stained green sweater I'd seen her wear a hundred times. I stood next to Fiona's brother at the funeral, slowly realizing that Grey had never revealed her relationship with me to anyone. As the priest drawled on awkwardly about how Grey had found peace and God, I couldn't help but be angry at him. *Found God?!* I didn't think Grey's actions had anything to do with *finding God. I would never know what thoughts had led to this. None of us would! How dare this man speak for her!*

I prayed that I'd find some way to live for her, to understand her, and to never end up in a casket this way. Since I had really looked up to her intellectually, I wanted to understand her actions desperately. I thought maybe she knew something I didn't know. But my art teacher from high school held me at her wake and said, "Tara. Trust me. You don't want to understand."

Numb

Grey's death, open-casket wake, funeral, cremation, and haunting journal entries *still* didn't stop me from wanting to escape. I still drank hard liquor every single night, took more pills than I needed, mentally tortured myself, and blamed everyone around me for not caring that I was hurting desperately.

I turned to self-harm, and then I blamed the people around me for it. Fiona was hurting badly from losing her best friend and was afraid that she would lose me as well. Before Grey's death, Fiona had spent what amounted to years of her life trying to convince Grey that she had reasons to live. She'd driven to Rhode Island to soothe Grey more times than she could count.

I was being nothing short of incredibly depressing, and Fiona finally told me not to talk to her anymore. I officially felt like I had no one who understood how I felt.

One night, I decided that I really was done. I called my abusive boyfriend and said my good-byes, but he was drunk and angry and said he didn't care. *Perfect,* I thought, *I don't care either.*

I took a box cutter that I'd swiped from work, and I hacked away at my left wrist, then went down my arm with blurry, tear-stained vision. I had kissed Raelie good-bye, written notes to all my loved ones, and shut off my phone. I put the hot water on in the bath and waited for it to fill up to get in.

As I sat mindlessly staring at the hot water slow-motion gushing into my dirty tub, the doorbell rang. It was my boyfriend. He did care, after all. After seeing me, he immediately started crying. Then, he started weeping and wrapped my gushing arm up in gauze, whispering, "What did you do? What did you do?" as he held me like a baby and I cried in his arms.

I stared at my arm in horror as blood filled the gauze and continued to trickle down my arm. I couldn't feel a thing.

Scars

I still have the scars on my left arm from this time in my life, and they are likely permanent. This is especially significant, because although I did start self-harming on and off my first year on lithium—at fourteen years old—at no other point before did I ever give myself scars or care if it was the last time I ever did it. I was hurting, big-time. And I was really pissed off that nobody cared.

This event led me to a new psychiatrist in New York, and to a prescription of a concoction of Xanax and Valium on top of the painkillers and mood stabilizers I was already on. My new doctor gave me very clear instructions: "Don't fill them at the same place. Without insurance, the Valium should only cost you just under fifteen dollars, so when you fill it, tell them that you don't have insurance."

I did as I was told. Sure enough, the Valium was cheap when I claimed I had no insurance, and I filled the Xanax for free at a pharmacy literally across the street. I would wait in one pharmacy for the Valium while the other pharmacy filled my Xanax prescription. Within twenty minutes I was on my way with both in separate bags. It wasn't until many years later that I realized that my doctor had given me those instructions because pharmacies *weren't legally allowed to be filling these prescriptions for me at the same time. I thought she had been helping me! Turns out, I wasn't supposed to be on these two drugs simultaneously!* **This concoction could have killed me!** Unknowingly, I took my Xanax and my Valium diligently.

This turned me full-zombie. Somehow in this haze, I realized that I had been working for a decade straight, either at a school I didn't belong in or at a job I despised. At just twenty-four years old I had already spent eleven years—almost half of my life—on medication. I had exclusively been in relationships with possessive people who hated themselves and always eventually hated me, and I had carried my family guilt from decades ago into everything I did, everywhere I went. I lied to everyone, including myself, to feel better about where my life was headed. The adage "Wherever you go, there you are!" haunted me, because I truly didn't like myself. The future looked pretty bleak.

Catalyst

The one positive thing Grey's death did was propel my desire for change. I had been to more funerals than I wanted to remember. I had lost more friends at a young age than I could have ever expected. In four years of high school, I lost over ten different friends to deaths ranging from suicide to heart surgery to unexplainable aneurysms. A young girl in my neighborhood accidentally hung herself on a swing. Death crawled around everywhere.

In my two years at Bennington, I went to five funerals. The most unbelievable to all of us was the beautiful girl who had fallen out of a window during a dance class. That was her last moment on earth. Everyone was devastated. That really struck Bennington hard, especially since just a few weeks earlier there was a car crash during a weekend drive home. That student lost her life too. A boy from my theater class hung himself in his room a few months later. Losing one student in such a small school was enough. I had lost three classmates in a year. After that, I went home for field-work term and never looked back.

But losing Grey was very different. I had loved her tremendously, and was overwhelmed with guilt that one of my best friends had taken her life just blocks away from me instead of picking up the phone and calling me—or anyone. Even though we had all been really depressed for a decade or more, I never, ever thought she'd actually kill herself. It's still hard to believe.

The last time I had seen Grey, in fact, was at another friend's funeral, and *even that had been déjà vu.* We'd been to too many funerals together. I had been to too many funerals and wakes, I'd been on too many depressing car rides, I had drunk too much alcohol, I'd stumbled around on too many late nights, I'd been hungover and stressed too many mornings. I had given too much of the wrong parts of myself to the wrong people, I had been sick for too long. I was tired of it all. I was done with it all, and I knew dying wasn't the way out.

"Anyone who has ever succeeded in any human endeavor will tell you that he learned more from his failures than he ever learned from his successes. If he's being honest."

—Tavis Smiley (1964–Present), American Author,
Outspoken Equal Rights Advocate, Philanthropist

Self-Empowerment

This prompted my first self-empowering decision: I broke up with the abusive person I had spent all those years trying to please, with absolutely no guilt whatsoever. At this point, I was becoming so selfish, so absolutely consumed in my own misery, that I didn't even care anymore that I was alone. *Being alone,* I thought, *has got to be better than being with someone who doesn't care about me.*

Breaking up with him wasn't triggered by finally understanding how this relationship had negatively affected me, although I wish I could say it was. After Grey died, nothing changed. My soon-to-be ex had absolutely no empathy for what I was going through, despite losing a parent just months before we started dating. I was truly just so exhausted I didn't have any energy to fight with anyone anymore, and I couldn't get through a single conversation without fighting with this person. One night I called him and laid it out:

"We don't belong in each other's lives," I said. "I love you a lot, but this hasn't been healthy for either of us. I have to let you go."

His response wasn't productive. He was mad, bitter, told me to go fuck myself. When I asked him, "Don't you even care about Raelie?" his response was clear, in no uncertain terms, that he did not give a shit.

Even though he didn't respond as I had hoped, I made sure, from that point forward, that I exerted a certain degree of care and sympathy with all my relationships. I knew, eventually, I would find someone who responded just as lovingly as I did. This, in fact, turned out to be a very valuable lesson: I will forever know when to turn the corner in a relationship. I will always know when I have grown apart from someone I love, and have to continue on my own path. I'll always know when to leave.

Turning the First Corner

I haven't talked to him one time since that day, and I didn't just break up with him. I broke up with the idea of accepting a toxic relationship in my life. Just a few weeks after breaking up with this toxic relationship idea, I started coming off my medication. Medication was possibly my most toxic relationship.

I did this cold turkey, meaning one day I woke up and decided I was going to stop taking everything—a daily regimen of Lamictal in the morning, Xanax and Valium as needed throughout the day, slapping on (or my favorite, very toxic method, chewing) a fentanyl patch for my pain, taking four Celebrex or eight Flexeril for my muscle spasms, whatever I felt like for my migraines, and then a Seroquel nightcap before bed to properly pass out. . . .

That morning, instead of doing my normal numb-out routine, I woke up, collected all of my medication into a big black garbage bag, and stuck them under my bathroom sink.

There, I thought. *It's done.*

Little did I know . . .

The Big Dose

I wanted to start over. I wanted a healthy body and to work with a clean mental slate. I wanted to feel things again, the way they were *supposed* to be felt—something I hadn't done in over a decade.

I had experimented with not taking my medicine in small doses before, but I had never actually committed to it because the withdrawal side effects were so frightening.

If I didn't take Lamictal, for instance, colors around me quite literally changed back and forth from deep saturated hues to less vivid ones. I would look up at a tree, and the green leaves would start to turn a vivid green, then a vivid purple-blue. I'd blink, and it would become normal again, and I'd be very relieved. But after a moment it would start its green-to-purple-blue pattern all over again. This alone convinced me I was crazy.

If I didn't take Lamictal in the morning, I would be driving to work and thirty minutes later I would look up and try to remember where I was going or where I was. Sometimes I'd even start driving to jobs I had quit *years ago*, like I'd lost years in my memory. Even if I recalled that I was driving to work, I'd have a hard time remembering where it was or what I was supposed to be doing that day. I'd leave work for lunch and halfway through my sandwich would have no recollection of what time I had left or when I needed to be back. I scared myself—a lot—but I did get through it. It's a little alarming to think that I drove at this time in my life—or that anyone may be driving on or coming off of many of these drugs.

Coming off Lamictal is also when I started to get very, very nauseous. I spent a lot of days in bed nauseous, sick, sweating, shaking, dizzy, and confused. My head was foggy and I couldn't hold on to any thoughts or keep any food down. I had to use a bedpan.

I got really, really sick in short order, but I think it's important to note that just a few weeks after coming off my first medication, *even though I was sicker than I'd ever been*, I truly started pursuing my dreams. I started meditating daily, I started focused on learning something new every day, I read books I had been putting off for years, and I started speaking openly with my family and friends. For the first time, I was learning to create a life around a concept that had always eluded me in the past: how to stop worrying.

I went through it. I started thinking clearly again, and reconnecting with people I hadn't seen in years. I realized a lot of things, among them that I had dated the same person over and over again, in different forms. I began to ask myself how I had gotten into toxic relationships to begin with, because I was determined to never experience anything like that ever again.

Sickness

An emotion is only wrong, bad, wasted, or negative when it's misused, and I had been misusing all of my emotions for years. *This had been my real sickness!*

After I realized this, and applied the idea to my life, I began to form healthy, honest relationships and focus on spending all of my days doing and working on *only* what made me happy. As you'll come to read, I immediately started to change my philosophy, my diet, my lifestyle, and my habits completely for the better. When I wasn't feeling sick, I spent every waking hour outside, exploring parts of New York I hadn't been to before or simply taking Raelie for a walk in a gross old stream, swamp, or trash pile by my house. These were legitimately the most scenic places.

I had big dreams, but they required big beliefs. Beliefs that I was capable, spiritual, connected, larger than life, worthy, talented, and could be successful. Beliefs that I could be happy, content, healthy, and no longer in pain or having daily panic attacks. I wanted the stress in my life to be gone. I wanted to be happy. I knew, finally, that I deserved happiness, and I was done holding myself back from it.

The Torturer

I was opening myself up to the idea that life might get to look different than it currently did. It might look closer to what I had always pictured, which was a hazy film of happiness. I still had no idea what my personal happiness looked like, but it felt freeing to be searching for it.

I knew there really wasn't any success without failure. I knew I was still learning from my mistakes, and I wanted to keep learning, hopefully without having to make too many mistakes in the future.

But a part of me knew I could turn back anytime I wanted to. I could slip back into old habits and old personality traits anytime I felt like it, so this mentality wasn't easy to start and the commitment wasn't simple to keep. I had never thought this way before, and I didn't exactly have role models at my personal disposal who had ever lived or thought this way. I was starting over, which I had never done before either.

Normally in the process, this is where we first start to give ourselves excuses. Excuses that we're too sick, too weak, or too unworthy to create the kind of life that we envy in others. Very few people want to actually acknowledge that they've made mistakes at all! That twinge of guilt or a bad feeling about ourselves holds us back from acknowledging when we've messed up. It blocks our path to everything good.

I let myself feel that guilt with no hesitation, all the time. Some days I let it absorb me completely. Y'know what I realized? It only lasted for a few moments longer when I *did* think about it than if I tried to skip over it completely. And then the crappy feeling would disappear *on its own*. I didn't need to force it to go away. My body *didn't want to feel bad.*

We can't carry around years and years of guilt or stress subconsciously. Our bodies actually won't let us do it, naturally. It's just plain uncomfortable for our souls and doesn't teach us anything biochemically. We have to keep reminding ourselves of what horrible, terrible, no-good, very bad people we are. We have to keep telling ourselves that the things we've seen or felt are too traumatic to deal with. We have to constantly remind ourselves how unworthy and uncomfortable and scared we are. And we have to do it over and over and over again for it to really stick.

I realized with a complete sense of wonder that the person who had been silently torturing and putting down my mind, my body, and my mental capabilities for my whole entire life . . . was *me*!

CHAPTER FOUR

MY NAME IS HERB

"Nature's first green is gold."
 —Robert Frost (1874–1963), American Poet,
Nature Lover, Four-Time Pulitzer Prize Winner

Okay, so I was my own enemy. I accepted that, and I was ready to change. Nothing I had done before had ever worked, and I wasn't okay with spending God-knows-how-long trying to sort my life out on my own. I wanted to get well *now* and permanently. But I had one last, triumphant excuse!

I had absolutely no idea what "being ready" to change my life really meant for me because I had barely lived, barely faced my emotions, and barely done anything different than what I had been doing for *years*! I'd never been off medication before, and had absolutely no role models for this kind of mental shift or life change. I knew I needed to rely on myself, and nature was there to provide me with some really useful aid that just didn't come in the form of pills or other people.

I started my research. I picked up some natural remedy books that had been sitting on my bookshelf for years, and I began to read. My research was simple, and I found my first herbal solution: vitamin D.

Vitamin D

I knew multivitamins had never really done anything for me, and that if I wanted to really get well, I'd probably have to start taking just as many supplements as I had taken pharmaceutical drugs. Since I was getting very ill and even brushing my teeth left me dry heaving and gagging for ten minutes, this seemed like a totally impossible task. So I was essentially replacing not taking pills with taking *different*, maybe even *more* pills. *Great.* Daunting or not, I knew I'd never really know until I tried, so I headed to my nearest pharmacy and picked up some vitamin D.

Vitamin D was the first supplement that I incorporated into my life, and it was the spark that ignited the fire.

After about two weeks of taking 500 IUs four times a day of D vitamins (starting in the morning and taking my last ones right before bed) I saw very real improvements. It helped me clear my thoughts, organize them, and really began to improve my mood overall. I became less brash, more kind, less judgmental, and had a cheerier attitude about everything I did. These multiple amazing results from this one vitamin inspired me so much that I started to research more natural remedies.

Investment

Americans spend more than $300 billion on prescription drugs every year, and nearly half of all adults have taken one prescription drug in the last month. However, I didn't know a single person who had a "daily vitamin regimen" or any kind of vitamin plan to treat their ailments. No doctor had ever suggested this kind of treatment to me either.

Women are prescribed—and take—more Rx drugs a year than men, and nearly a third of the population regularly uses one or more prescription drugs. I had spent a lifetime's worth of money on prescription medication, but I could barely justify purchasing *more than one* bottle of vitamins.

That's because as much as I researched, I still wasn't inspired *to invest in myself*. I had at least fifty tabs bookmarked on my computer for supplements I really wanted to try, but I could never bring myself to *actually purchase any of them*. What kind of an investment was I making in myself? *Not much,* I realized.

Making a self-investment, whatever that is for you—whether it's finally going on that run, booking that cabin in the woods, buying those yoga classes, making that cup of tea instead of coffee—is the first step to changing your own destiny.

The Whole Idea

Many of us reach a certain point in our road to wellness, and then just stop. This is the most common problem: we get good results from one practice, or two, but we're reluctant to invest in the whole idea. The Whole Idea is the new formation and creation of ourselves as better people in better jobs doing better things with our lives. From the most desperate situations to our most accomplished days of success, it is important to continue to keep the Whole Idea in mind and to see how it changes, adapts, and shifts with our lives. Even if we are completely comfortable, it is always encouraged to reflect on how this idea came into play to manifest this for us.

"One person with a belief is equal to ninety-nine who have only interests."

—John Stuart Mill (1806–1873),
British Philosopher, Self-Improvement Enthusiast,
Influential Contributer to Social Theory and Politics

Especially in circumstances where everyone around us is doing something totally different than we are for their health, it's hard to believe in our own healthy decisions, even if we've experienced positive results. We become resistant to concentrating on our life choices, and worse yet, we experience tremendous self-denial about our own success.

This is where conviction becomes a very powerful tool. Choosing challenge over comfort, adventure over safety, or visibility over invisibility is an investment in ourselves.

Motivational speaker Zig Ziglar put it best when he said, "You'll never make it as a wandering generality. You've got to become a meaningful specific."

Becoming a *meaningful specific* means making a name for yourself, whether it's at home, in a classroom, during a social event, at a lecture, or where-*ever!* It means something different for all of us, depending on where our journeys are taking us, but it's profound for every life. Your meaningful specific may be pottery, math, crafts, parenting, stocks, writing, dancing, singing, or connecting with people or animals. Whatever it is, our goal should be to nurture its growth, much like we do with plants, which incidentally are also here to help us grow and thrive.

Natural Nausea Treatments

The next thing I researched was supplements that cured nausea. I had finally given in and tried everything available over the counter or available by a doctor to rid myself of the daily shakes, dizziness, and hours spent being sick in the bathroom.

I wanted so badly to be able to work without getting sick, to live my dearest dreams, to apply all the insight I was gaining through meditation, to expand on the knowledge I was acquiring—intuitive things that I had only just been imagining a few weeks prior.

I had tried every single over-the-counter drug or drink claiming to cure nausea I could find. Each and every one of the remedies I ingested ended up "coming up" and I'd watch their neon colors swirl around the toilet bowl after I flushed it and immediately reach for my toothbrush. There *had* to be something natural that wasn't an artificial color, that didn't need to be drunk, and that didn't taste horrendous going in—or even coming out.

Digestion

Digestion often works in mysterious and complicated ways, and our gut is a gracious host to over a thousand different kinds of bacteria. Anything from our imagination to our sense of smell can trigger it; even traumatic events can have an effect on our appetite.

Probiotics are microscopic, bacterial organisms that work to replenish the beneficial bacteria in our gut in order to improve digestion and body function. Probiotics are beneficial to your intestinal flora, supporting the body's ability to process food. When the digestive tract is healthy, it can easily weed out all the crud that ends up in our bodies, like processed food, pollution, toxins, chemicals, and bad bacteria. Probiotics aid the digestive tract in its health, and have been shown to help everything from bladder cancer to UTIs to acne.

I finally ordered acidophilus probiotics off the Internet. My closest option while I waited for my order was kombucha, another suggestion that had come up in my research.

Kombucha

Kombucha is a fermented, effervescent drink made from a symbiotic colony of bacteria and yeast (a SCOBY) and an herbal tea. It was known as the "Immortal Health Elixir" by the Chinese around two thousand years ago and has been credited with improving digestion, strengthening the immune system, aiding in weight loss, detoxifying and cleansing the body, and has played a role in cancer prevention.

Kombucha contains probiotics, B vitamins, enzymes, and a high concentration of acid. I started drinking kombucha daily, and eventually ordered a SCOBY and tea set off the Internet and began to make it myself at home. It was easy, and in about two weeks' time I had an entire gallon of delicious homemade brew in the fridge.

Drinking kombucha daily really did begin to help my nausea after only a few days, and if I drank it diligently and meditated on schedule, I only felt sick in the mornings, and only when I thought of the impending day of work. Stress, it seemed, triggered my nausea too. Despite all these triggers, my frequent projectile vomiting turned into dry heaving with the occasional upheaving, and I found my first ray of hope.

Changes

All of these changes I had made in my mentality, my philosophy, my personal acceptance, and my attitudes had really started to show their improvements in a few short weeks. I wanted to be a stronger person than the one I was. I no longer wanted to be sensitive to what other people thought of me. I wanted to feel a strong, indelible sense of self. I wanted to find my true purpose. To be the bohemian, beautiful, healthy love warrior I always wanted to be. I wanted to travel, to experience life, to grow, to move ahead in my personal growth. I was tired of being bored, frustrated, constrained, and dull. I wanted true mindfulness. I wanted to know I wouldn't quit when life got tough. I wanted to know myself, the way I'd known myself just over a decade ago, before starting lithium or Lamictal. Maybe even better than I knew myself back then.

When my probiotics came in, I saw more changes immediately. The first day, I took four 200-mg acidophilus tablets, and have never wavered since; sometimes I would take more, just in case, but never less. I took them every day right before bed. One morning, I woke up, took a shower, brushed my teeth, and realized while combing my mane that I hadn't thrown up once.

Prior to this, I had been throwing up every morning of every day for *six months*. I cried of happiness right then and there, with the curling iron around the base of my hair. My digestion was better, my skin was clearing up a bit, and I could think with way more clarity within a few weeks of a daily probiotic regimen.

Herbs to Curb Worry, Stress, Insomnia, & Anxiety

It was around this time that I started to consider more herbs to help with certain emotions that I was trying to control with meditation; guilt, anger, and resentment were big ones. I had an unexplainable rage that had begun when I started taking lithium at thirteen years old. I was very sensitive to other people's emotions and certain things would just set me off. Not only did I have panic attacks every single time I had a fight with family members, I was also affected greatly by other people's moods. If someone around me was in a particularly bad state of mind, or spoke in a certain tone that could only be described as harsh or terse, I would respond just as curtly and find myself in a panicked state of mind.

This feeling created a physical emptiness in my stomach that no drug, drink, or other person could ever soothe. It was as if I was very full, and yet still needed a gallon of anything from the nearest food chain.

I was consumed by rage and anger toward myself and others, but I wanted to learn to forgive and move on for good. First and foremost, I wanted to forgive myself, but I also wanted to truly forgive other people whom I felt wronged by. These thoughts were keeping me up at night, and I was suffering from severe insomnia again.

The only time in my life I even had any remote control over feeling was during my daily quiet meditations. I knew there had to be other ways to fight this battle.

Natural Valium

Valerian has been used as far back as the first millennium—that's right, circa 100 BCE. Back when Trajan ruled the Roman Empire and when Marcus Aurelius declared himself the "Protector of Philosophy" (*ooo la la!*), both Hippocrates and Galen prescribed the valerian herb as a sleeping agent for their patients. The name itself comes from the Latin word *valere*, which means to be *strong and healthy*.

I found valerian at Whole Foods in New York City, and picked it up because the box was labeled FOR NERVOUS TENSION, which was the closest thing to describing my symptoms that I'd *ever read*. Little did I know that natural valerian may work similarly to Valium, one of the drugs I had come off of so recently. It would never have occurred to me, because valerian feels *absolutely nothing* like Valium.

I started by taking valerian in tea form. It was the first herb that I tried for my insomnia, but it did a lot for my anxious moods too.

Valerian tea is prepared with the roots of the valerian plant (*Valeriana officinalis*) and some hot water. It's known for its natural, side effect–free sedative qualities, its ability to calm the central nervous system, and its penchant for soothing aching muscle groups. Valerian has been used for hundreds of years for the treatment of insomnia resulting from restless thoughts or nervousness and anxiety. In studies, sleepiness and dream recollection seem to be unaffected.[3]

I had been prescribed drugs to help me sleep for years. Flexeril, a muscle relaxant, was one. It was supposedly for my muscle tension, but all it ever did was knock me out. I would often wake up before my eye muscles did, and spend the first five minutes pulling them open with my fingers and trying to get them to work. My eyes, it turned out, were still drugged up.

On Flexeril I would often wake up thinking, *When did I fall asleep, and what did I do before I did?* Complete gaps in my memory remained. I left it up to my partner at the time—the same one who had been hurting and manipulating me—to fill in the gaps. *Good luck, sister.*

There was also Seroquel, which I'd been prescribed at Bennington by the college psychiatrist. Labeled an antidepressant, Seroquel had made me so exhausted that I missed several dozen classes in college from sleeping in. "My drugs cause drowsiness," was not an excuse my professors liked. At all.

Unlike these drugs, I liked the way valerian made me feel. It wasn't the relaxation I had always expected when doctors said they "had something for me to try" but a soothing feeling I had never experienced before. It didn't make me feel high or light-headed, just dreamy and lovely. It didn't knock me out either. I just experienced a mild, natural euphoria from the warm tea. I would often drink a few cups and take a long bath with Hima-layan pink salt and a few ibuprofens thrown in before bed. I found myself in much better spirits.

Other great herbs that are safe to incorporate into your diet for insomnia, anxiety, and worry are: kava, feverfew, hops, and lemon balm. These come in tincture, tea, and loose herb form and can be added in a variety of ways to your day to motivate and progress your wellness.

Herbs to Curb Pain & Promote Muscle Relaxation

My healing process for my back had, at one point, definitely regressed. When I was around thirteen years old, my mom decided to attend one of my physical therapy sessions for my scoliosis treatment. I had gone to these with Dad, who always sat patiently in the waiting room reading the newspaper while I worked through my exercises.

During a pull-up I was doing on the bar, my mom stopped the physical therapist. "Um," she said, and I could feel the nervous anger in her voice, "I think you're doing those *backward*."

"No, no," the therapist insisted. "This is the correct way."

"Excuse me," said my mother. "But **no**. It *isn't*. Her curve goes *this* way," she said, gesticulating, "and you're twisting her spine *that same way* when you do this exercise."

The therapist left to check my X-ray, and came back to say that my mother was right. However, the therapist insisted, this was the first day they had done the exercise wrong. I quickly denied that, since I'd been doing these monotonous exercises for over twenty-four months. Dad, my mom, and I left in a huff.

Needless to say, I never went back. My mother was absolutely furious, and she made a huge deal about it. It *was* significant: it meant that *over the course of the past two years I had been attending physical therapy, they had been making my back worse, instead of helping it.* The place closed before we could file a claim.

Now, a decade later, I was no longer taking all the pharmaceutical painkillers, nerve blockers, and muscle relaxers I had relied on for years to mask my incredible discomfort. The pain was still very much real and I needed to find an alternative solution.

The Epsom salt baths I took while drinking valerian tea relaxed my muscles, which were starting to feel like small rocks in my back. These baths were also my favorite places to meditate. With my body submerged underwater, I could see myself clearly for who I truly was: a bored, frustrated, constrained soul who had been dulled by past experience and the idea of fitting in. I had been selfish and lazy, and I was tired of my old self. I would often bring a book in the bath with me — a quiet read soaking in salt suds was the first real luxury I afforded myself.

In the bath I could finally relax my body and concentrate. I had many visions of a life I hoped for, where I was pursuing my dreams in a sunny place.

The valerian experiment was so encouraging, I decided to try some other natural remedies for the same symptoms. I figured that since I had taken so many drugs for so long, taking something natural for the same ailments *couldn't hurt.*

The next herb I tried was *Lavandula angustifolia.* I read this attractive name to myself a few times while waiting in line to buy my first fragrant baby lavender plant. This was my virgin attempt at gardening of any kind, and I was a little skeptical of my ability to keep this cute, sweet-smelling little thing alive. However, I had read that lavender was amazing for sleep, grief, pain, anxiety, stress, and fear, so I was determined to at least *experience it,* and buy flowers from the Internet if I had to in the future. I put the little guy in front of my bedroom windowsill, watered it daily, prayed that it would grow, and picked a few flowers off every day for tea.

As it blossomed, I started drinking a combination of valerian tea mixed with some flowers from my lavender plant, which I often talked to and sometimes even apologized to. I plucked off each petal delicately and placed them into a tea catcher. I'd often fill it back up three or four times, making sure I consumed every last therapeutic drop. I drank this tea tonic with a few drops of honey as many times as I wished each day. Sometimes I even sipped on it all day in small doses.

It undoubtedly helped my debilitating migraines, which disappeared after just a few days of drinking this tea, and have never returned. The persistent kidney and bladder infections that had lasted for over a decade, kept me bedridden, and turned into septic infections time and time again became less and less frequent, and eventually stopped popping up completely.

I also added lavender flowers to my bathwater before bed for an extra boost of aromatherapy and hydrotherapy. My hydrotherapy involved immersing myself in a hot bath followed by turning the showerhead on cold for a few minutes while I meditated. The cool water over my face, scalp, and body while submerged in hot water was invigorating and lovely. This soothed my aching muscles and calmed my nerves.

Chamomile

Since I was sensitive to caffeine from an early age, I was already familiar with chamomile, which is used to make one of the most common caffeine-free teas on the market. Chamomile contains anxiolytic properties, a fancy way of saying it naturally inhibits anxiety.

Chamomile also has anti-inflammatory properties. And boy, were my muscles in-flamed, up-flamed, bi-flamed, uni-flamed, and ohmyfuckinggodmakeitstopplease-flamed! There were so many nights when I just wanted someone to cut my back out and replace it with a new one. I could barely raise my arms in the shower to wash my hair from sharp arthritis pains, and I often put my head upside down to shampoo as a less torturous compromise.

I had spent over a decade taking drugs to resolve or mask my pain instead of finding healthy ways to relieve it. Once I stopped using the drugs and could finally feel what was *really* happening inside my body and the kind of pain I was *really* in, my days were totally agonizing. The barometric pressures of New York were definitely irritating my inflammation, I was sure of it. As autumn approached, I spent many days crying in a scorching hot bath, feeling crippled. I remembered doctors telling me I may be paralyzed or hunchbacked by the time I was in my thirties. At twenty-four, I *felt* paralyzed on most days, and was starting to believe I actually was. My muscles cracked like bones. The pain was agonizing, overwhelming, and consumed all of my thoughts. On some days I even wished for the uncomfortable gasps between projectile vomiting I was getting coming off my medication, over the debilitating pain that my scoliosis, arthritis, and inflammation caused. The discomfort came from my very bones.

Chamomile helped soothe my discomfort straight at the source. Chamomile extract is shown to stimulate osteo-based cells, lubricating joints and inhibiting bone loss. This was crucial for treating my arthritis.

Chamomile also promotes restful sleep patterns, manages diabetes, promotes menstrual cramp relief, boosts immunity, and soothes the stomach.

Melatonin

I'm really not the kind of person who needs to read a hundred good reviews on something before I buy it. If it's changed one person's life, I'm pretty much sold on the idea of trying it. I'm a sucker for a good story. So when a dear and talented friend told me about melatonin, I was sold immediately.

He told me that he couldn't sleep. Thoughts, duties, bills, girlfriends, dates, work, living, the government, the wars—all plagued him on a daily basis. He had no idea how to function in a world that he thought of as hopeless. He didn't want to have kids because he didn't want them to be born into a world like this. Despite being attractive and well-off, he was single for four years and had never had a deeply meaningful relationship. He hadn't read a single book since high school, at least not the whole way through.

He told me, "The idea of self-reflection was meaningless to me. In fact, I scoffed at it. I also scoffed at happy, fulfilled people. I sure didn't understand happiness, and I sure didn't feel like I deserved it! Melatonin changed all of that for me! Within a few weeks my whole life was different. I *thought* differently. I have a relationship with someone I'm proud of. I started at a job I love. I'm becoming who I wanted to be all along. You should try it!"

That same week I was waiting in a doctor's office for blood test results, and I picked up a magazine. In it, I found an article for "sluggish" people. *Sluggish* was a word I identified with *a lot*. It suggested taking melatonin for sluggishness or for people who weren't sure what to do with their lives. I read it, resonated with it, researched it, and I even considered buying it on my phone right then, but didn't. In fact, I completely forgot about it.

A few weeks later I was in a grocery store, and they were doing a demo in the store with free samples. When I looked closer, I found myself smiling ear to ear. It was melatonin—the same brand that had been in the magazine! I immediately put two quick-dissolving melatonin items in my cart, and began taking them immediately when I got home. I think I even opened one in the car, but then read it needed to be diluted, and didn't have any water.

Within a few weeks, just as my friend had said, I was making incredible life decisions that I had always been afraid to make before.

Melatonin is found in humans, plants, bacteria, and fungi, and it is the most fundamental and universal hormone that we know of in the evolution of cellular life. Melatonin has faced Western controversy because it is a naturally occurring hormone—not an herb or a plant supplement (unless you count the fact that it's also found in plants).

What I wanted the *most* was self-control. I accepted that I had become what I thought about all day long, but I hadn't yet mastered *how to think differently*. I desperately wanted to start thinking differently so that I could have new thoughts, form new patterns, engage in new behaviors, create new actions, and ultimately, become a new person. My thoughts of "I'm too old," "I'm too sick," "I'm too weak," "I'm too tired," or "I just can't" were consuming me daily, and I was trying to rid myself of them for good.

Over time, I started to take four small tablets of melatonin in the morning and four before bedtime, which dissolved on my tongue and tasted like peppermint. (To be fair, that's 'cause I got the dissolving, peppermint-flavored kind. It doesn't do that naturally.)

When I started taking melatonin, my sleep patterns immediately improved and my thoughts seemed to be rewired for the better. I looked forward to taking melatonin each day. It didn't give me any immediate feeling of wellness, but a good sense of well-being did lovingly creep in after a few hours starting on day one. I loved the idea that I was *finally* taking something in pursuit *of truly caring for myself*. That thought alone was extremely effective and reinforcing for me.

Human production of natural melatonin decreases with age. Our melatonin levels are most regular at around three months old. I was almost certain that at three months old, I probably wasn't being cared for properly. Since I was exposed to drugs and alcohol in the womb—which I knew I was—I may not have produced a normal level of, well, *anything*. I wondered if I *ever* had produced a normal level of melatonin *at all*.

In *Autobiography of a Yogi*, Yogananda writes, "Man has allowed his consciousness to identify itself almost wholly with a frail physical body, requiring constant air, food, and sleep in order to exist at all." This felt very true for me. I needed an explosive boost.

Melatonin is also known as the "timekeeping" hormone. Coming off birth control and finally "seeing" myself for the first time had reminded me that I wasn't getting any younger. I had been staring twenty-five right in the face, without a single day of self-reflection or a single life goal accomplished. I was trying my damnedest to be the best, most self-reflective, most healthy, beautiful person I could be, and all I felt was sick. Before starting melatonin, I had stopped writing altogether.

A study was conducted in 2009 at the Université Pierre-et-Marie-Curie in France. Scientists found that melatonin had significant antiaging effects on shrews, animals that begin to show signs of aging around twelve months, due to a loss of circadian rhythm in their activities. This study showed that melatonin slowed the signs of aging for the shrews at around three months—a significant relation in respect to their life span. It was also noted as an antioxidant and antidepressant.[4]

After a mere few weeks of taking melatonin, my migraines were absolutely gone! With a regular sleep pattern, a good night's rest, and no reason to keep the curtains drawn, I already felt much better, even while going through withdrawal. Looking back, I think I can attribute this small miracle in part to the melatonin increase: despite the severe curve in my neck, which should place my head at a sideways angle, I only experienced a dull aching in that area.

But don't take my word for it. At the sixty-fifth annual meeting for the American Academy of Neurology, it was shown that "3 mg of melatonin was more effective than a placebo and had efficiency similar to a 25-mg pill of amitriptyline, a common sleep aid."[5]

The melatonin showed lower rates of daytime sleepiness and no incidence of weight gain, which is a common side effect of many prescription drugs. Another study published in *Neurology* found that two-thirds of patients taking 3 mg of melatonin nightly experienced a 50 percent reduction in headaches per month. The duration and intensity of those headaches also significantly decreased.[6]

Thoughts to Help Pain

My new herbal regimen had improved my digestion, decreased my pain, and helped me sleep better, but it still didn't eliminate my problems altogether. I knew coming off the medication had a huge hand in my daily dry heaving and violent sickness, but there had to be another root cause to the nausea that I was missing.

Ultimately I narrowed this down to a combination of the way my spine curved and the grief I still felt over Grey's death. I felt unbearably more nauseous on days when my back hurt the most, during times I had depressing ideas about my future or days when I missed Grey terribly. Anytime I panicked, nausea set in.

Every therapist I saw about getting over Grey's death was totally dismayed that I wouldn't take any drugs to help myself. It turned me off to grief therapy, so I took matters into my own hands. Instead of thinking about grief as something I was "getting over," I started to think about it as something I was *getting through*. I began to realize that grief was another inevitable journey I was on, and if I could become familiar with the different twists, turns, pitfalls, and pathways on the way, it was a journey that might not be so hard the next time I inevitably went through it.

I started listening to every lecture and reading every book that I could get my hands on. I immersed myself in the positive aspects of my situation, whether it was at the library, book in hand, with headphones in, on a walk, or on forums for people coping with grief. I reread the Tony Robbins books that I had read so many times as a kid, when I was adjusting to a new living situation. I watched his free videos online and took every single recommendation. I even read and reread inspired blog posts from contemporaries who had been lucky enough to attend my mentor's lectures. I downloaded old episodes of *Oprah*, and watched the TV mogul interview people going through many situations similar to what I was facing, garnering massive applause for their bravery. I wrote letters to all of my deceased friends, including Grey. I spoke to her, and spoke to other people about her. I was totally receptive to other people's ideas about spirits, angels, and the afterlife.

I took my first-ever therapist's amazing advice again: I shared my story with others. I thought about a single idea a lot until I knew I had come to a true understanding, and then I would let that thought go. I focused on the positive elements of Grey's life, and mine. I was grateful. Grateful to be alive, and grateful to have known her. If I had a certain sad memory, I would constantly switch to focusing on all of our treasured memories together. I sent prayers to her soul, to her family, and even to a "past" her—the one who thought grabbing that gun was the answer. I sent love to everyone. I started to take the focus off of myself and my grief and put it back onto other people. I put the focus on Grey and her struggles and her poor, hurting parents. I sent healing thoughts to Fiona, who I knew was still struggling.

When I caught a train on time but just barely, when I heard good news, when something in my life completely synched up, I said a silent, "Hell yeah, man." When good things happened, I thanked her. I felt like she was guiding me. I could feel her presence with me all the time.

I had often pictured myself checking into a psychiatric ward when my grandparents passed away. They were my rock and I didn't know what I would do without them. I wanted to prepare myself, so I wouldn't resort to drastic measures when it did happen. I knew that losing both my grandparents was inevitable. Losing one's loved ones is inevitable.

So I tried to imagine what could have possibly pushed someone I loved so much to do something like that—to take her own life so violently. That way, no matter how bad things became, I could stop myself from doing the same thing.

The answer, I realized, was not just pain, but the hopelessness. The *will to live* determined everything. I knew this because I had been in very much the same place. I had the scars to show for it.

I had been physically, mentally, and emotionally exhausted. I had felt stuck and hopeless. I had thought about ending my life.

I had even tried to. And I never wanted to be there again. I knew prescription drugs had never helped Grey, and was finally realizing that they'd never helped me either. I was on a renewed search to find a natural cure for the pain. I wanted to be my best self, and I didn't want to settle for anything less.

My thoughts were the catalyst I needed for overcoming my physical pain. It was all connected. The idea of succeeding in wellness finally became more important than all of my other ideas. I knew nature had a whole medicine cabinet of its own: ancient herbs, tonics, cures, and secrets that had so far been surprisingly easy to find. I knew that my thoughts determined absolutely everything, but so did what I was putting into my body. Without a healthy body as my foundation, my mind would never have what it needed to *stay well*. It was one thing to get well, but to *stay well* I had to not only form new thoughts, I had to adopt a whole new lifestyle.

Natural Painkillers

GINGER

Ginger was one of the few herbs that I discovered I already had in my kitchen cabinet, and one that I already really loved using while cooking. I was super excited when I first read that ginger has been used since the dawn of Ayurvedic history, and records show its use in Greece around 200 BCE. Ginger tea was described by the ancient Koreans as "the beverage of the holiest heavenly spirits," a fact that piqued my interest quite a bit at the time. Confucius wrote back in 500 BCE that he was never without ginger when he ate. In 77 CE, Dioscorides recorded ginger's warm, softening effects on the stomach. The ancient Chinese used it for scurvy.

Myself? I had been using it for digestion, putting small pieces into my tea catcher along with the valerian, lavender, and chamomile. But I started throwing ginger into everything I made to up my intake for pain management. I had begun a raw diet—mostly because I had to; I couldn't really *eat* anything solid yet. I ate mostly smoothies, salads, nuts, mushrooms, and very simple fruit- or veggie-based meals. This had nothing to do with weight management, since I've always been small and was certainly not trying to lose any weight. It had to do with the fact that not only could I not really digest anything very well, I truly wanted to start over.

I had eaten like crap my whole life. You know what I'm talking about: rewarded with fast food, dessert, ice cream and persuaded with chips, soda, burgers, fries, ice cream, and milk shakes at every turn. I had also grown up in New York, The Ancient Land of Pizza and Bagels.

I donated my microwave and cut out anything processed, all fast food and all junk food. This was not easy, but it made a lot of sense to me once I did my research. If I bought everything myself, it was cheaper, safer, and easier to eat it all at home. Leftovers were simple. This super-convenient method prompted my entire life's work in nutritional wellness.

I started to put ginger in all of my smoothies, all of my salads, soups, juices, every cup of tea, and I also took it in pill form (just in case). On my particular kind of pain—including rheumatoid arthritis and pain from my bones and muscles— ginger can work miracles. In fact, a University of Miami study concluded that ginger extract could serve as a substitute for common NSAIDs (or nonsteroidal anti-inflammatory drugs) like aspirin and ibuprofen, with no harmful side effects.[7] Ginger reduced the pain of osteoarthritis in patients by 63 percent over a placebo. Georgia College & State University in Milledgeville also reported in the *Journal of Pain* that a few tablespoons of ginger a day helped ease muscle pain caused by exercise. It works on a cellular level, because it contains anti-inflammatory, anti-ulcer, and antioxidant agents, as well as small amounts of analgesic properties.

To feel pain, your body must produce pain signals. It does this by sending quantum, subatomic responders to the brain. While ibuprofen is a common pain remedy, it has no effect on our *natural* production of pain producers or the natural inflammatory chemicals in our bodies, such as cytokines. Cytokines are immune-regulating substances that can have inflammatory effects and are often linked to pain.

Also, much like the rest of the coping mechanisms I had adopted previously, taking ibuprofen for my pain didn't teach my body anything. It wasn't teaching my body how to produce, say, its *own* painkillers, its *own* natural response system to pain, or even its own *threshold* for pain. It was just masking it, confusing my neural pathways and delicate cellular receptors into thinking there *was no pain* when there *was pain.*

Ginger extract has been shown to reduce cytokines—those little inflammation-causing buggers—in comparable amounts to prescribed drugs, and was just as effective at reducing pain levels. Dr. Krishna C. Srivastava, a world-renowned researcher of the therapeutic effects of spices, found that ginger is actually a superior pain reliever to ibuprofen, because it works by breaking down *existing* inflammation and acidity in the fluid within the joints. It accomplishes this by blocking inflammatory compounds, such as prostaglandins and leukotrienes.[8]

Within a week, I saw major effects on my pain level. By the second week, I was convinced that the added ginger was truly helping. Immediately upon even smelling ginger, I would stop over-salivating, which is how I knew it was truly working. Over-salivating and breaking out into a cold sweat were the first and very telltale signs I exhibited when I had attacks of major nausea.

TURMERIC

Turmeric boosts more than your circulation—it's been used for over four thousand years, has been proven to exhibit anti-inflammatory properties, and is widely used for joint problems, arthritis, and immunity. Turmeric is part of the ginger family, and is high in anti-mutagens (anti-mutagens 13 and 14, to be specific), which drive off the really nasty new cancers caused by chemotherapy or radiation.[9] I stumbled upon turmeric — of all places — through my family.

My aunt had gotten to the point in her joint pain where raising her arms was sheer agony. This slowly inhibited her work, and after a while she decided that retiring was a better option than straining herself as a nurse, even though she loved it tremendously. After trying a medley of prescription and OTC medications, she decided to try something she had seen on television. Turmeric, a woman on an episode of *Dr. Oz* had said, had *cured* her arthritis.

My aunt bought turmeric and started incorporating it into her life tentatively. She added only a few pinches to her cooked dinners. After a while, she added a few more pinches. Then, she started putting it in her salads. When she got used to its raw taste, it went on her cooked meals *after* they had been fully prepared, as a final touch. Soon, she started drinking raw smoothies of fruits, veggies, and turmeric.

One night, in bed, she reached for the remote control to change the channel. While staring straight at her arm, Auntie was astonished. It was raised above her shoulder! She screamed for her husband to come in the room, and raised her arm again and again. "Look!" she shouted happily. "It *moves!*"

She attributes this recovery 100 percent to the turmeric. This started her on a drastically new lifestyle of her own, but for me, it meant, "Okay . . . maybe I should try it."

I had long associated turmeric with Indian culture and had been hesitant to try it in my day-to-day diet because it reminded me so much of dinners I made with my ex. Doused in curry, turmeric, garlic, and "harsh spices," these medleys of veggies were primarily dishes we threw together because we were poor, and they were cheap and flavorful. But they were also classic dishes from his culture and the smell reminded me *a lot* of his house. Turmeric had made up many of our dinner nights at home.

After we broke up, I stopped flavoring my meals with turmeric altogether. But after hearing my aunt's testimony, I decided to rid myself of this association. Turmeric could potentially save my life, and I couldn't let the fact that it reminded me of someone who was no longer in my life ruin it for me. I tried turmeric over and over again until the taste no longer reminded me of him. Each time I ingested it, I thought only about my path to wellness and my growth, and forced myself to keep him off my mind. I wanted to change my approach to this food, maybe all food. Much of it had great stresses and anxieties attached to it.

For instance, many of the fights I'd had with my grandparents had occurred at the dinner table. It seemed like we couldn't help but jump down each other's throats about something every night, and I was constantly either leaving the table or finishing my meals alone because someone else had left in a huff. Not long after I moved out I realized that this association made me angry around dinnertime, and even a little stressed out and nauseous having dinner with others.

The goal was to rewire my brain so that when I smelled turmeric—or anything that reminded me of anyone else—there wouldn't be negative triggers any longer. When I truly let it, turmeric gained an extraordinary place in my life.

It also had an extraordinary impact on my livelihood. Eventually after trying it raw time and time again, the only thing turmeric reminded me of was my own kitchen. Like my aunt, I also started tentatively taking it internally, pinching it into my smoothies, adding a dash to my soups, throwing a tablespoon into my breakfast in the morning. After a few weeks of incorporating turmeric into everything I ate in larger and larger doses, I really began to feel a change.

Not only was my nausea even more at bay than it had been previously, my joints felt more fluid. I could move in ways I had not been able to move before. My shoulders, which had given me agonizing pain for years, were finally functioning close to normal; my lower back pain was only happening nightly or if I strained it a lot.

Turmeric has stayed in my diet ever since, and if anything, has increased and had more dramatic effects over time. It's a daily part of my wellness regimen, and has completely replaced all of the scary pills I used to take for pain and inflammation.

GARLIC

Allium sativum. It produces year-round crops. Egyptians worshipped it. It's been used as currency. Entire genres of folklore have been written about it. It's been touted as an aphrodisiac for ages.

Those might not be your first thoughts about pungent, tear-inducing garlic, but this raw plant contains allicin and diallyl disulfide, naturally occurring antioxidants that have been studied to help a number of ailments, from heart disease to cholera, from cancer to typhus, from yeast infections to arthritis.

I love garlic, and was totally willing to give up fresh-smelling breath for some pain relief and healthy joints. I started just chewing a few cloves a day while I was cooking. It gave my stomach a quick release of acid that seemed to calm my nausea, and it had incredible effects on relieving my arthritis too. Garlic also made its way into my baths. The smell was actually quite soothing. On days of severe pain, I would simply toss a few cloves into a steaming tub and relax as the aroma calmed my tension and provided incredible hydrotherapy.

I also drank garlic, much like I did with ginger. Both of these plants are common in Chinese cooking, and I researched different methods of preparation. My favorite was straining garlic cloves in a tea catcher and sweetening the herbal tea with honey. If you have any kind of aversion to garlic, I'd recommend this as the way to get over the hump. Garlic has replaced some of the nastiest anti-inflammatory medications that I took, like Celebrex, Vioxx, and Flexeril.

SKULLCAP

I first came across skullcap while researching alternatives to valerian. The valerian was working really well, but I wondered if there might be another herb I could take in tandem for those super agonizing days of pain and restlessness.

Common in America, but also used in traditional Eastern medicine, the plant's name was finally coined by European settlers after the helmets worn by their soldiers: skullcaps. Skullcap (*Scutellaria lateriflora*) is a part of the mint family, and is a nerve sedative for conditions like hysteria, nervous tension, anxiety, alcoholism, insomnia, migraines, and epilepsy. It is similar to benzodiazepines (the family of drugs that contains Valium and Xanax—both drugs I had taken in the past). All plants in the mint family can be classified as super-plants for super health.

I started to take skullcap in tincture form before bed at night, adding some to my teas. It started working immediately, giving me a more relaxed attitude, better rest, a happier sense of well-being, and had an immediate positive impact on my pain. Skullcap is believed to lower blood pressure, blood sugar, and cholesterol, which all may have contributed to the feeling of euphoria associated with taking the herb. Always the skeptic, I would go a day or two without skullcap just to see what happened. I fell into a sluggish, deconstructive pattern every time. Again, I would add skullcap to my teas at night, and fall asleep restfully within minutes. I'd wake up rejuvenated in the morning, my joints and bones fluid, my mind immersed with ideas and plans.

Skullcap is also very useful for treating withdrawals, which I was certainly going through. I had never thought of myself as a drug addict before, but every day reminded me more and more of what I had seen my mom go through when she had decided to stop doing heroin. The sweats, the cravings, the incredible pain in every single muscle and joint in my body were almost more than I could bear. If it wasn't for all of my terrible past experiences, I may have even checked myself into a hospital. I considered it many times.

Instead, I took more herbs. The skullcap also helped with my bladder infections, PMS, depression, exhaustion, muscle spasms, anxieties, compulsive thoughts, empty feelings, and confused rationale. They all slowly disappeared. After drinking skullcap with my teas, I felt so calm and relaxed, that the last thing I was doing was second-guessing how I felt about myself, my life, or my path.

Herbs to Curb Depression

ST. JOHN'S WORT

I had been "warned" about St. John's wort for as long as I had been on prescription medication. This is due to strong evidence that St. John's wort has a great effect on depression and pain management—just not the effect you would think.

The delicate yellow flowers of St. John's wort are used to produce tinctures, teas, and capsules full of natural medicine that's been proven to help ailments such as fibromyalgia, addiction, alcoholism, chronic fatigue, headaches, muscle pain, nerve pain, ADHD, menopause, obsessive compulsive disorder, seasonal affective disorder, HIV/AIDS, minor depression, hepatitis C, and inflammation (everything from muscle inflammation to bug bites!).[10]

Doctors are instructed to tell patients that this herb may interfere with their medications for *the same ailments that the herb treats.* On many of my prescriptions, there were often notes warning patients *against* taking St. John's wort, even though the prescriptions were for *exactly what St. John's wort is good for!* In fact, France has banned St. John's wort specifically because of the way it interacts with pharmaceutical medications.

What I had never been told in my pharmacological therapy was that neurotransmitters—that is, important cells that carry messages to and from the brain—need to receive certain signals from my body to deliver those messages properly. I had never been asked about my diet or exercise and had never been suggested supplements during therapy. I had never been educated about having a healthy body in order to have a healthy mind.

In order to think optimally, our brains need to receive important, naturally occurring chemicals that allow them to combat anxiety, overcome grief, or get out of a slump or depression. St. John's wort has actually been proven to keep more antidepressant and antistress neurotransmitters available for the body to use. Some studies suggest that it may naturally raise the levels of the neurotransmitters dopamine, serotonin, and norepinephrine in the brain.[11]

Honestly, I believed that St. John's wort did help me with all of these things, but most importantly to me, after incorporating it into my life, I suddenly had much better control over my plaguing, unwanted, obsessive thoughts. They ranged in subject, from the *why mes*, to the *I should have saids*, to the *next time that person does this I'lls*. These thoughts were truly nagging and entirely distracting. I'd be planning something lovely, moving on with my life in a big way—and then *bam!*—I'd realize fifteen minutes later that I was in the middle of a rage of angry thoughts about my past. This had frustrated me entirely, because I really wanted to move on and I didn't want to sit around ruminating about problems that truly didn't even matter. I had too many amazing plans and goals to be focusing on instead!

St. John's wort also helped relieve my PMS, or the premenstrual symptoms that occur for some women during their time of the month. Mine came about two weeks before and then continued until my period was over. It stole about half my month, every month. Cramps, mood swings, hormonal breakouts, crying spells, and the like were all very common for me and I was so tired of them. I felt absolutely awful, but I had always believed that it was natural to feel this way, and that it was maybe something that I would simply have to accept as part of my life. After all, that's what everyone around me had done. I had seen girls get days off from school and work *just for this reason* plenty of times in my life.

The truth was, *I really didn't want to accept being in emotional and physical agony for what would eventually become half of the rest of my life.* After coming off birth control and all of my other pharmaceuticals, my body was way out of whack. I was getting my period on time every month, but the pain it caused was unlike anything I had felt before.

About two weeks after taking St. John's wort along with the other herbs—valerian, chamomile, ginger, garlic, skullcap—I got my period and suddenly realized I had no symptoms! I hadn't even realized that it was coming, even though it was on time, because I barely had any bloating! The crazy mood swings, crying spells, emotional roller coaster, terrible pain, and bad cramps had completely vanished! I was over-the-moon happy, but still skeptical.

"We should not be extremists in any way, but should adopt whatever methods of healing are suitable according to our conviction."
—Paramahansa Yogananda (1893–1952),
Indian Yogi and Guru, Psychic, Kriya Yoga Teacher

Herbs to Cure Aging, Acne, & Skin Troubles

These herbs were certainly making me feel better, but one big problem still remained: my skin.

The worst part of my withdrawal ordeal besides my nausea was my skin, which started breaking out uncontrollably. I had battled pretty terrible acne as a teenager and it didn't go away until I started taking birth control at sixteen.

My first few weeks into taking birth control my skin became radiant and clear, freckly and youthful. I battled a zit or two here and there, but I also never really gave my skin a second thought. I never wore makeup, but I also never diligently washed my face at night or in the morning. In college, I'd go a few days without washing my face. I didn't have the best skin in the room—it never made anyone envious—but it was never *bad*.

Almost immediately after I stopped taking birth control, I started developing hard, painful, cystic acne along my jawline, chin, neck, and mouth. This was particularly embarrassing for me, considering my aspiring profession as an actress and singer.

Cystic acne is the type of acne that causes abscesses produced by infected oil ducts under the skin and can occur from genetics, hormonal imbalance, drug withdrawal, stress, an unbalanced diet, or, in my case, all of the above. Gross—I know! Not only is it super painful and sore when touched, it's impossible to hide with any amount of makeup. In fact, foundation and cover-up always made it worse for me, reinfecting my skin and really highlighting the awful bumps along my face, jawline, and chin.

Unaccustomed to this mess on my moneymaker, and totally desperate, I did what anyone who gets whiteheads all over their face does: I unskillfully popped them. This is the first time I realized that whatever I was dealing with on my face in my twenties was *not* what I had battled in my teens: these suckers *wouldn't drain* (even *grosser!*). Not only did my feeble attempts to aestheticize myself leave me with much worse inflammation, but the holes I gave myself after picking my skin would take weeks to heal, and then leave awful scars. I wanted to hide more and more every day. I was at a total loss; my self-esteem was down the toilet. *Was my skin*, I thought, *doomed to be bad forever?*

DIM

I was at a complete loss over what to do about my skin. Photographs from that year show rough, bumpy, dehydrated skin, early wrinkles, bags, crow's-feet, and an acne-erupted jawline. My acne was also "underneath the skin"—sometimes never coming to a head but staying craterous, painful, and unattractive all over my face. I was also extremely oily by my nose, cheeks, and forehead, but very dehydrated everywhere else, including my body. Redness appeared, and bouts of psoriasis on my arms and on my legs every single time I shaved. Parts of my skin looked red and rough. This did very little for my self-esteem.

I also experienced strange things since coming off my birth control: unexplainable hunger that never left no matter how much I ate, severe bloating, heavy bleeding that led to anemia, and a very decreased sex drive. It was actually starting to sicken me to even be touched, which was unlike my personality and very upsetting to me. Whether this was hormonal or a combination of withdrawals and my new low self-esteem, it didn't even matter to me.

I made an appointment with a dermatologist, and begged her to put me on Accutane. I was absolutely miserable, and often got depressed or felt suicidal *just because of my skin*! She compromised and gave me a prescription for minocycline, which I had been on quite a bit as a teenager.

Minocycline is an antibiotic prescription medication used to treat bacterial infections, including the kinds that cause acne. I had first been prescribed this medication back when I was twelve and thirteen, and it had worked mildly for a short period of time. My dermatologist then had warned me that often the body becomes tolerant to the medication, and sometimes the effects of the antibacterial medication will naturally wear off. This is exactly what had happened: within two weeks my acne reappeared, and the oral medication never worked again.

I had a feeling that this medicine would do nothing to tackle my severe adult acne if it hadn't worked on moderate acne a decade ago, and after second thought and some deeper research, I realized that I really *didn't* want to go back on *any* kinds of medications, especially ones like Accutane or minocycline that can cause moderate to severe depression—exactly the thing I was trying to *prevent*! I never filled my prescription. Minocycline would be another bandage: a medication taken to treat the current symptoms, but not to address the real cause.

Instead, I started researching natural causes and treatments for hormonal acne, which is what my dermatologist had told me I had. If the problem that I had was hormonal, I knew that an antibiotic wouldn't be the solution. Antibiotics are for infections, not hormone imbalance.

Hormones are chemical messengers secreted through the endocrine glands. They travel through your bloodstream, tissues, and organs to relay messages about growth, metabolism, body temperature, reproduction, sexual function, and mood. Insulin, for instance, is a hormone. It regulates the amount of sugar in your blood. Too much or too little insulin can lead to either diabetes or hypoglycemia, or even be fatal.

Plants also have hormones, such as auxins, which are responsible for their behavior and growth. Hormones are especially important during puberty, because they begin to determine when and how your body starts to change. For women, they also play a role in our mid-twenties and then again in our early fifties, a period in life also termed menopause.

Forty-five percent of women in their twenties suffer from adult acne. That's almost half of the population. In my search for natural treatments, I came upon the universally recommended things like vitamin D (which I was already taking diligently), zinc, selenium, and magnesium—all supplements I had tried in the past with no huge improvements, although they all did make me feel better overall. Then, I started losing my hair. This was the huge breaking point for me.

Every time I took a shower and brushed conditioner through my hair, clumps of it would fall out. I was horrified. I felt sicker than ever, even though I was finally trying to get well.

Then one day, completely by accident, I came upon what is now my go-to skin-saving solution. I was sent an email about broccoli (true story) that held the answer to all of my skin problems: a substance called DIM.

Diindolylmethane, or DIM, is a plant substance formed in the body through consuming cruciferous vegetables, like broccoli, cauliflower, sprouts, and cabbage. Scientists think it acts much like estrogen, but also like an estrogen regulator, metabolizing the "bad" estrogens, balancing hormones, relieving PMS symptoms, and acting as an anticancer and preventive cancer measure. DIM, indeed. I felt absolutely dim for not knowing anything about this supplement before!

DIM is produced when the body breaks down indole-3-carbinol (that compound found in cabbage and other cruciferous vegetables mentioned above), which is used for the treatment of fibromyalgia, tumors, abnormal cell growth, and lupus. Some people use I3C to "detoxify" and "cleanse" their bodies, which it certainly did for me, even though that wasn't my original intention or even my original experience.

My first DIM supplements were shit. That email about broccoli was an educational mass-spam for a supplement called Estroblock, a brand I was intrigued by immediately. After some research, I purchased them on a small hope. They claimed to "block" my estrogen levels and therefore regulate my hormones: a very simple and very convoluted way of explaining how DIM works and exactly how it was supposed to be healing my body. Estroblock didn't have bad or no effects, but it certainly didn't have the effects I was hoping for.

That is, until after a month into it. I did some research on the brand that I had bought, and it turned out a lot of women had been having the same issues. They "kind of" saw improvements, but not the ones promised to them. Finally I found one review that recommended a supplement from Nature's Way called DIM Plus. It was sixteen dollars. At a third of what I was currently paying, I almost cried. Also, the reviews were glowing. Women said it had changed their lives, reversed menopause, cleared their stubborn acne, revived their sex drives, and so forth. I purchased it immediately.

Within just a few days of taking this kind of DIM, I saw miraculous improvements in my skin. Within a week I noticed my first difference. My mornings spent dreading looking in the mirror for the rough bumps under my skin and unsightly whiteheads were slowly becoming less and less frequent. When I woke up, my skin was actually clear, and getting clearer every day! Then, the bumps stopped appearing altogether! In fact, they only happened sometimes, like if I forgot to wash my pillowcase or my face before bed, or ate a ton of dairy.

At first I took the recommended dosage—two capsules at 120 mg each—but after these minimal improvements I switched to four 120-mg capsules daily, taken in the morning with my smoothie. This is when I saw dramatic, drastic improvements overnight.

The first morning I woke up after switching to this double-dose regimen, my skin was legitimately smooth. I bawled happy tears, and ran my hands over my face again and again and again. I couldn't believe it! It felt completely renewed—like what I had always expected would happen after going to an aesthetician getting a chemical peel, seeing a dermatologist, taking prescriptions, or applying the thousands of acne treatments I had tried. I was so happy; I felt more like myself, like I was finally getting my life back! But I was also immediately frightened at the thought that, like minocycline, Proactiv, OTC medications, and things I had tried in the past, this solution would be temporary.

It hasn't been temporary. Three years later and my skin is as clear as ever. It gets better every day. Along with a healthy diet and nightly meditations focused on picturing clear, clean, healthy skin, taking DIM supplements has been nothing short of miraculous for my skin and my life.

Other supplements and herbs that I take in conjunction with DIM for my skin are omegas 3, 6, and 9, black currant, olive leaf, and evening primrose oil.

Healthy Skin Meditation

Sit up straight with your feet planted firmly on the ground.

Breathe In slowly through your nose, picturing your skin lit up from the inside, out.

Breathe Out through your mouth slowly. Picture all of your toxins, pollution, and chemicals being released from your body.

Breathe In slowly, picturing your light getting brighter and brighter.

Breathe Out: I release my darkness.

Breathe In: I accept healthy skin.

Continue this exercise for as long as you wish, but try it for at least seven breaths. Open your eyes and greet your happy skin.

Cancer-Fighting Herbs

With all the carcinogens we are exposed to on a daily basis, I wanted to make sure I was putting my body in the best position to fight and prevent the disease as possible. My family had a history of cancer: my mom had a scare with it, as well as my uncle, my aunt, and many of my neighbors. Floral Park, New York, my hometown, had 135 cases of breast cancer alone in the four years from 2005 to 2009. That was 49 percent above the expected rate. I was determined to ward off this predator before I faced it.

ASHWAGANDHA

Ashwagandha has reduced the rate of breast, central nervous system, colon, and lung cancer cells and is great for osteoarthritis, anxiety, coughs, and colds.

Ashwagandha is an adaptogen, an agent that creates biological effects that promote balance in the brain and body. Much like, say, Valium is supposed to, ashwagandha changes the neuron receptors in the brain. Unlike Valium, however, it is totally natural and it enables GABA molecules—the ones that control fear and anxiety—to connect easier, organically inhibiting stressful feelings.

Ashwagandha is the lubricant for your GABA receptors, the very same receptors that Valium and Xanax were supposed to be using to alleviate my anxiety. When GABA activity is increased, blood pressure drops, heart rate and breathing slows, and we become deeply relaxed.

Over 40 percent of our synapses work through GABA receptors. So, why wasn't I just prescribed ashwagandha or other GABA precursors by my doctors, instead of pharmaceutical drugs?

Many people are. It is one of the most powerful and useful herbs in Ayurvedic healing. Frequently used as a ginseng in India, it's in the same family as the tomato, and bears cute little red fruit about the size of a raisin.

I began to take ashwagandha as a tincture, nightly. It's also available in tea form, and regular capsules. Immediate benefits have included a killer immune system, and less soreness in my muscles. I am noticeably less stressed, my body feels cleansed, and I am kinder and much less nervous. A great way to take it is to drink it with herbal tea.

Stress Prevention Tea

Step 1: Boil your favorite herbs in a tea catcher.
Step 2: Add four drops of your ashwagandha tincture, leaves, or a full capsule. Let it sit for a few moments, stirring gently. Add cinnamon, turmeric, cacao, or anti-inflammatory herbs as necessary.
Step 3: Say out loud, "I am thankful for my health."
Step 4: Enjoy proudly! With every sip you are on your way to becoming your own wellness warrior!

RHODIOLA

Rhodiola is one of those miraculous herbs I wish someone had told me about a very long time ago. The rhodiola plant has been shown to decrease tumor activity by increasing the body's resistance to toxins. Makes sense, right?

A range of antioxidant compounds are found in *Rhodiola rosea* that prevent free-radical scavengers from attacking your precious cells. This also makes it an amazing agent for skin care. Oral use of rhodiola inhibited tumor growth in rats by 39 percent and decreased metastasis by 50 percent![12] It also improved urinary tissue in patients with bladder cancer.

Too much or too little serotonin is linked to everything from SAD to clinical depression to schizophrenia. Rhodiola is very helpful in combating depression because it both lubricates and enhances the transport of your body's serotonin precursors. Serotonin has been proven to help your body perform functions including promoting smooth muscle contraction, focusing on your everyday behaviors, normalizing blood pressure, regulating pain and body temperature, and achieving mental ease.[13]

Rhodiola has also been shown to improve cardiac problems caused or aggravated by stress. It decreases the amount of steroids and hormones released during stressful times. The abnormal presence of these hormones is what subsequently raises blood pressure, cholesterol, and potassium levels.

Rhodiola seemed like a perfect cancer-combating, free-radical-fighting herb to begin my "cancer-preventive" journey. It was good for my skin, good for my moods, good for my stress levels, great for my heart, and tasteless. Hopefully it was kicking some cancer ass too. I began to take it in tincture form, adding some to my tea, and also taking capsules of vitamins at night. Overall, I was feeling better, I immediately acted better, and pretty soon I realized I was truly *getting better*.

The Healing Tea Ritual

Step 1: Boil your favorite herbs in a tea catcher. Pour the herb water into your favorite teacup.
Step 2: Add four drops of your rhodiola tincture, herbs, or capsule. Let it sit for a few moments, stirring gently. Add cinnamon, cacao, or anti-inflammatory herbs as necessary.
Step 3: Say out loud, "I am drinking for my health."
Step 4: Repeat, "I am drinking for my health."
Step 5: Enjoy proudly! With every sip you are on your way to becoming your own healer!

Changes

The only regret I have ever had with herbs is that I didn't start taking them sooner. They've changed my life entirely—from giving me the energy that I need to pursue a tough day of work, to aiding me in the good night's rest I lacked for years. I often think, *If someone had told me about this years ago, I could have saved myself a lot of trouble!*

Once I started incorporating these natural little buggers into my life, I was convinced that herbs were truly where it *was at* for my wellness. When nothing else worked, they alleviated symptoms that I had been plagued with for years! Although I had felt very hesitant about trying herbs at first, once I got over that and started taking them, started realizing why they worked, why they were the intuitive and natural

solution, and began seeing the results, I knew that it was the right move.

In fact, I started to feel more confident in almost *all* of my decisions—a feeling I had never felt before. This eventually became one of my character traits, one that people would come to know me by, and one that would be very handy in my future success.

"He who asks questions cannot avoid the answers."

—Old Proverb

Your own wellness journey with herbs will be entirely your own, and I am so excited for you to embark on it! Incorporating even some of the herbs mentioned in this chapter along with a healthy diet and exercise routine can begin to help you on your own path to recovery, wellness, and the healthy body and mind that you seek.

PART TWO:
STAY WEIRD

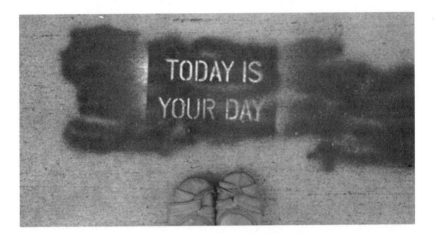

CHAPTER FIVE

THE DREAM

"All true scientists know that the true laboratory is in the mind, where behind illusions, they uncover the laws of truth."
—J. C. Bose (1858–1937), Bengali Polymath, Physicist, Biologist, Spiritual Botanist, Archaeologist, Science Fiction Writer

While sick and bedridden, I dreamed that I'd someday soon be completely content, active, medication-free, pain-free, in my own house, traveling the world, thriving with Raelie in a sunny place. I wanted Raelie to have space to run, and I wanted a little house to call my own. I wanted to spend my days doing what I loved. I longed to live out some of my most impossible dreams every day with people I admired, changing the lifestyles of people around me for the better, just by being myself. Staring at the ceiling, gulping on some lemon water, my throat raw from vomiting, I thought, *I want desperately to do this without the help of any pills, people, doctors, or shock therapy.*

Since I decided to recover, this has become my daily mantra: not to cover up the pain, but to face it. Not to hide from my fears, but to tackle them. Not to avert from others, but to converse with them. I started to focus on turning pain into meaningful healing, turning dis-ease into ease. I focused on making something out of nothing. I continue to do this each and every day.

What prompted me to start this journey was not my first wake-up call, not my past, not Grey's death, not staring into Raelie's food bowl as ants ravaged her food and my pad. It was not my toxic relationship, my breakup, my listless job, or my dingy New York apartment. No, those just inspired the first day I decided to stop taking the medication. But none of those events were the breaking point that really solidified my mentality.

The breaking point came a few months *after* I was off all the pharmaceuticals I had relied on for years. I was sick. Really, hopelessly, helplessly sick, and I was lying in bed for hours with Raelie until she smelled like my body odor. I was constantly shaking uncontrollably, dizzy or vomiting, until I couldn't breathe and was gasping for air.

So, I thought, this *is detox.*

Raelie's Intervention

Detox was horrific. It ebbed and flowed, which was the hardest aspect. I never knew if I was going to wake up sick, dizzy, or throwing up (although I could pretty much guarantee that it would be one of the three). The panic associated solely with not knowing when I was going to feel better again made it worse. I spent many hours just hoping, praying, and wishing that someday this would all be worth it.

A few times a day I crawled outside to take Raelie out to do her business. Once, while trying to take her out, I was so weak that I lost my footing and my grip on the railing. I fell down the flight of stairs leading up to my apartment. Not a small flight of stairs either. I missed about thirty or thirty-five steps on the way down.

I woke up in a pool of blood. I had bit my bottom lip through almost completely. Raelie woke me up with kisses on my face, but she soon went from whining for me to respond to wagging her tail and licking my face as I woke up. I looked at her, half slurring, "Baby girl . . ." as blood spilled out of my mouth. I felt I may have hit a new bottom, literally.

When the bleeding didn't stop within an hour, I called a cab to the emergency room. I ended up getting sixteen stitches right in the ER, which I can feel with my tongue to this day. I was also pumped up with antibiotics. It turned out *I had infected my own mouth* when I bit through my lip, probably from however long I was lying there soaking in my own blood. *Glorious.*

While I was getting stitched up, I could hear an eight-year-old girl with anorexia and a man with a gunshot wound who coughed through every word, both speaking to different doctors within earshot and only a curtain between all of us. I gagged through my conversation with the doctor, excusing away my nausea. It didn't matter; the doctor never asked what was wrong with me. This *still* wasn't my breakthrough.

The Last Straw

I spent the following days sick in bed, staring at the ceiling asking, *"Why me, though? Why the hell am I, after all the tragedy and heartache and crap I've already gone through, not getting better when I am trying my damn best to do the right thing? Did I lose everything for nothing? Will I really be able to make money doing something that won't make me sick? Would medication even do anything if I took it again? Should I just take it again?!"*

The first few weeks that I started to clear my head, these disempowering thoughts crept into my mind all the time. Soon enough, they became the triggers to my sickness. Whenever I focused on negative thoughts, I would almost always end up with my face over the toilet bowl. I wondered if there had been a link all along to my anxiety and my extreme nausea.

It occurred to me every once in a while to just take a Lamictal to feel better. I had relied on this medication so heavily that even a few hours of not taking it would have incredible effects on my mind and body. I'd started to see things in hyper-color again, like someone had turned the contrast up. I'd become deeply confused about where I was or what I was doing, even in normal day-to-day situations. Countless times during high school and college I had declined invitations to go out on dates or go to parties or sleepovers after school because I didn't have my Lamictal with me. The worst withdrawal symptoms I ever had were when I was coming off of the mood stabilizer that had "started it all" for me.

I had a lot of thoughts about taking "just one" Lamictal pill. Just *one* wouldn't hurt me, and then I'd be able to sit up, get up, move, speak, and function without the terrible weakness, dizziness, nausea, headaches, and oversaturated vision. *Just one* and I'd have my life back.

One day, when the withdrawal symptoms were especially excruciating and these thoughts very prevalent, I zombie-swaggered into the bathroom and opened up the cabinet under the sink, taking out the garbage bag full of Rx bottles that I had thrown together when I decided to come off all my prescription medication. It was full of not only pills that "had worked," but pills I had been prescribed that definitely *didn't work*, ones I'd only taken once or twice and then discarded—totaling what added up to almost a hundred different bottles. I kept picking up bottle upon bottle looking for the lamotrigine (the generic name for Lamictal that appears on the label). Valium? Nope. Xanax? Nope. Celebrex? Nope. Seroquel? Nope. Flexeril? Nope.

I discarded them one by one before I found the Lamictal bottle and emptied two blue, dust-covered pills into my palm. I filled up a glass of cloudy, lukewarm New York tap water and opened my mouth. A ritual I was so familiar and comfortable with.

And then, something truly remarkable happened.

I *stopped*.

My mouth still open, I stared at the pills in my hands, and I gasped in a hoarse whisper.

After three weeks of not taking any medication for anything, I finally realized *exactly* what I was doing. Taking "just one" Lamictal *wouldn't be* taking "just one." There was *no such thing* as "just one." There was only a lifetime of them, or nothing. Either I felt like I needed them, or I didn't.

Whenever I inevitably decided again that being at the mercy of a pill to "stabilize me" or "get me through" things was not what I wanted with my life, I'd be right here once again. Sick, debilitated, and debating. In three more weeks, or two more months, or three more years, this is where I'd be.

I'd be counting the amount of pills still in the bottles, nauseous, and hoping I have "the right one" for whatever ailment, uncontrollable emotion, or terrible feeling I was facing that day. It felt *way* more helpless and *way* more hopeless than feeling sick. I *knew* withdrawal sickness was temporary. Relying on a pill to control my emotions? That was something else. The realization of exactly what that was, that was my breakthrough.

Lifelong Helplessness

Whether it was the amount of medication filling that black garbage bag, whether it was the sight of those blue pills I had not seen for weeks after seeing them every day for a decade, or whether it was the weight of the garbage bag when I finally picked it up and brought it curbside, somehow, I realized that my mind and my body had been succumbing to lifelong helplessness. And I wasn't going to accept that in my life anymore.

This was my real breakthrough. At the time, I didn't even recognize it as the amazing thing it was. I had completely solidified my decision to change my life philosophy.

Any talent that we are born with eventually surfaces as a need, the calling we're all given eventually gets too loud to ignore, the voice inside of you that knows right from wrong sometimes can't shut up. I had given into this idea completely, without even realizing it. While it wasn't easy, it felt incredibly rewarding. I wanted to live my dreams. I wanted to be well, I wanted to feel normal— whatever that meant. I wanted to at least use some crazy thoughts for good and constructive projects.

I realized again that I had two inner voices that were always battling each other: the voice that knew what the right thing to do was, and did it, and the part of me that knew what the right thing to do was, and did the opposite. It was The Voice again. The good news was that no part of me couldn't recognize that I definitely needed to change. I wanted the part of me that knew the right thing to do, and did it, to be the only voice I heard ever again.

From here I looked for other ways to cope.

Coping

I realized that before these last few weeks in my life, every action I took, every job I had, every class I sat in, every paper I wrote, every journal entry, every kiss, every problem I faced, every relationship, and every friendship had been at the mercy and suggestion of a pill I took. Not one single person I had ever loved or known had ever asked me *if I actually thought I was crazy.* No one stopped to question if I *should* be taking medication to help any of these ailments—pain, anxiety, mood swings, depression, bad decisions, bad grades, or family issues. They only debated *which* medications I should be taking to solve these problems.

No one had asked me if I felt like I *was* bipolar. They just labeled me bipolar as a child and walked away. "Problem solved!" they thought. "Now all we need to do is adjust her meds!"

A childhood, adolescence, and adulthood spent on so many drugs gave me a high tolerance for pain. I had to be on death's door to ever get anywhere near a hospital, and often was. I had been plagued by unusual and frequent bladder and kidney infections, which popped up every three months starting just weeks after beginning lithium and became frequent at the age of fourteen. These infections were resistant to a lot of antibiotics. During an oral at-home treatment, I got a septic kidney infection and I worked with it throbbing for a week. This eventually left me in the hospital for two weeks.

Emotions

Strong emotions can override pain signals in the body. Examples include when we feel invincible, when we "must" work through an illness, when a mother is trying to save her child, or when a

121

soldier fights on in battle after sustaining an injury. Our tolerance for pain doesn't rely on the amount of pain itself, but on a host of chemicals in our bodies called endorphins and enkephalins, which were discovered in the 1970s.

They're in a family called opioid peptides, which are produced to release a morphine-like substance that originates naturally from within the body. The main function of these peptides is first, to release natural painkillers to the brain, and second, to produce a feeling of happiness or euphoria. These little guys also serve to prohibit the transference of pain signals to the brain *to begin with*. But, depression, anxiety, or an awful diagnosis often discourages these good endorphins from being released. This explains the rise and fall of pain, even when we are experiencing acute symptoms of an underlying disorder, such as when I was working through my septic kidney infection, or when people live with cancer for years just to die only days or weeks after they're diagnosed by a doctor.

Conversely, if we are telling ourselves with conviction we are truly well, and *we are living it*, we can thrive for years with our dis-ease without giving it any power. When we focus on the positives our body releases more endorphins, giving us a natural tool to fight our diseases and illnesses.

Endorphins have an added bonus when they naturally occur: they're nonaddictive. Unlike much of the pain medication I had been prescribed to relieve my symptoms, releasing endorphins naturally *never* had any negative or withdrawal symptoms for me. By choosing to focus and float on the positives, I was able to help my body release natural endorphins. If I was sad, I would make myself laugh. Whether this was in the form of just laughing until I couldn't anymore, or specifically turning on an episode of *Family Guy* for half an hour, I was determined to no longer dwell on depressing thoughts.

People who say making yourself happy is a harmful distraction aren't truly believing in their happiness and well-being. While there's no evidence that a "prescription of natural endorphins" would work across the board for everyone, the power of suggestion during placebo trials has been very intriguing regarding this matter.

In study after study, when a patient is given a placebo (a sugar pill or a dummy drug that has no chemical effect on the body) but are told that they're taking a painkiller, an overwhelming percentage (generally between 30 to 60 percent) of the patients experience pain relief, sometimes equivalent to that of morphine.[14]

Morphine isn't chemically identical to endorphins, though. In fact, *morphine seems to pale in comparison to the complex method in which our natural endorphins create pain relief.* Exercise, yoga, acupuncture, meditation, chiropractic, and hypnosis are all valid forms of pain relief based on endorphin release, but we can create these within ourselves as well.

Control Your Pain

Our thoughts have a vibration similar to light, sound, and solids. They can be measured.

The ability we have to control our pain is based on a principle called *nonlocality*, a term quantum physicists coined in the 1980s after dozens of physicists found hard-evidence-experiment after hard-evidence-experiment to support it. Nonlocality is the ability of a quantum entity (an individual electron) to influence another quantum particle (another electron) instantaneously over distance despite no exchange of force or energy.

It proved everything: that your energy affects my energy, that our energy affects time and space, that we all affect one another. It proved that no matter how far apart electrons become separated, a connection is *always* retained. This shattered the very foundation of physics at the time.

This is because it scientifically suggests that, even on a larger scale, *everything* is connected. We are connected to our minds, which are not located in our brains as we originally thought, *but in fact located throughout our bodies.* When you get depressed, your skin cells also get depressed. When you get depressed, the

people around you connect with that energy, and are also suscep-
tible to getting depressed. Each cell interacts not only with each
other, but with each and every other thing in this universe, all the
time.

All the saints, all of the prophets, all the influential icons that
we know of, were just people like you and me. Jesus, Babaji, Yogananda, Moses, Saint Anthony, Abraham, Gandhi, Mother Teresa,
Martin Luther King Jr., John Lennon—all walked among us. This
is profound to me.

We all have the same capabilities of these living saints. They all
told us so. They all promised enlightenment, gave the tools, and
reminded us that *we're no less divine than them*. Without even
considering ourselves divine, every single day we are tapping into
the same source that *created* our pain and limitations, which can
conversely be used in order to *release* them.

Divinity

Imagine what we could do if we *did* consider ourselves Divine? A
human brain that changes its very thoughts into chemical signals
that affect the body every moment *is*, in essence, *amazingly divine*.
We all have the ability to do this incredible thing, making us all
amazingly divine.

Indians have a word for this: *Brahman*. From the Sanskrit word
for *big*, a Brahman is an invisible field, an unchanging reality that
is amid and beyond the world. It is also called *Sat-chit-ananda*,
meaning "being-consciousness-bliss."

Brahman meant nothing to me the first time I read it. It literally
didn't mean anything. I imagine to a New Yorker, it rarely does.
It was total and complete nonsense. I stared at the word and actually sounded it out multiple times. I read and reread the meaning,
trying to apply it to my life.

Eastern culture had always completely eluded me, and I felt
a certain separateness from these kinds of foreign words and
their hidden essences. I again gave into the idea that maybe I was

dumber than I thought. Honestly, I don't think Brahman is something that's supposed to be understood the first time. I didn't get it until weeks later.

A Friend of a Friend

In my stage of reconnection, I found a good friend named Stace, whom I hadn't seen in a few years. Every time we hung out we always had fun together, but Stace was also always on and off pharmaceuticals and making five-year plans to move to California. Ten years later, she was still in New York, rummaging through my jewelry ("Ooo! Shiny!") and questioning my desire to stay off pharmaceuticals forever.

We became fast friends again, and I confided to Stace about the horrible symptoms I'd been having from withdrawing from medication. She encouraged me to get out of the house, and that same week she introduced me to someone who would become one of my greatest teachers and allies, a boy named Henry.

Stace showed up to my apartment with a bottle of wine and a fistful of Valium, and brought me to a recording studio to play photographer for her boyfriend's band. Someone was filling in for the bass player during the photo shoot.

When I first met Henry, he had a paper bag over his head, because he looked nothing like the guy who played bass. The paper bag had a smiley face drawn on it, which I silently snickered at the entire time. I was giddy and amused. I was having *fun* again.

I watched the band properly rock out, snapping away. When the set was over, only one person came up and introduced himself to me. It was the boy with the bag on his head!

"I'm Stamos," he said in a Midwestern drawl, sticking out his hand. I took it. He went on to explain his nickname to me. Before he could finish, I interrupted (still a bad habit at the time).

"I get it," I said, smiling. "Like John Stamos." He looked just like the guy! Uncle Jessie in the flesh!

His eyes lit up.

"Yeah," he said. "Like John Stamos."

"I'm Tara."

I immediately felt that this boy had made his way into my life for a reason, and I was truly struck by how nice and interested he was. I spent the rest of the night wondering why I had stayed in such a suffocating relationship for so long when there were so many amazing, interesting people to meet.

I played my own music for Stamos, whose real name was Henry—a soulful R&B tune called "Visual Exchange" that I had just shared online. He dug it a lot, and we started making music together that very week, forming a band we named Hindu Doggie in the first month of knowing each other. We'd spend hours in my apartment, making trippy sounds with MIDI keyboards and guitar as I sang my heart out over these chords and wrote the first set of lyrics I had written in years.

Henry also handed me a life-changing book the first week we met one another—*Autobiography of a Yogi*, by Paramahansa Yogananda. It had an Indian person on the cover whom, at first glance, I thought was a woman, and as I dug in, it started to really change my life. Henry also told me one of the most important things I had heard:

"You're not crazy."

It was by swallowing this sentence for the first time after sharing my story that I had my first real mental shift. It wasn't just about not going back on medicine for something I may or may not have, *it was about completely abandoning all the previous beliefs about myself that I had carried with me all of my life.*

It wasn't that I needed someone else's validation to convince me, but hearing those words from someone else meant something larger: Henry was the first new friend I had made since coming off my medication. Everyone else I had seen was from my past, and knew me as a crazy person with all these different diagnoses. But this person? He was new. And he had a totally different perception of me than everyone else!

"Fatigue, discomfort, and discouragement are merely symptoms of effort."

—Morgan Freeman (1937–Present), American Actor, Film Director, Narrator, Political Philanthropist

Doing Your Best

I was still working at a job I really despised, but I wasn't messing up at it quite as much. I had inspired talks with my co-workers, even though I had to leave for the bathroom every fifteen minutes or so to throw up. But no one gave me a hard time. I started making plans, and reading *Autobiography of a Yogi* religiously. It became my bible (no offense to the Bible, which was my original bible!). I found myself underlining every other paragraph. I pictured myself walking the same beaches and wandering around the same grounds where *Autobiography* was written. I started really saving my money and opened up a savings account for the first time in years, where I put three-fourths of every paycheck. I was becoming more inspired and responsible by the day.

I also picked up *The Alchemist*, by Paulo Coelho, another book Henry recommended. The idea of *Maktub* was totally enthralling to me. *Maktub*, a word used throughout *The Alchemist*, means, "It is written," as in, everything is bound to happen exactly how it does. No outer force can interrupt or disrupt it. There are no mistakes. *Maktub*, in essence, is your written destiny.

I was determined to live my destiny. Every day, no matter what I was doing, if something inspired me, I stopped and wrote it down. I also did this each and every night before I went to bed. I woke up excited about my dreams and goals, and it gave me a lot of inspiration to work on getting better. I continued my breathing exercises, mantras during my meditation, and centered the ideas in my mind around self-healing and self-love.

I encourage you to do this in both small and large ways: leave yourself loving notes on your calendar, on the fridge, taped to the bathroom mirror, or in a place you know you will see them every day. Set a happiness alarm! I had a mantra I really loved taped to my wallet and my desk at work: *Just keep doing your best, and your best will get better.*

I had never believed in anything so fully before. It was in reading *Autobiography of a Yogi* that I rediscovered Brahman. It finally meant something to me: it meant becoming consciousness, becoming "being," it meant being aware, and a promise of bliss. An old Indian proverb says, "A man who has not found Brahman is like a fish who has not found water." I had very much felt like a fish who had not found water. A breathless being, flopping around helplessly on a deserted shore. Totally out of my element. *Brahman was exactly the connection and the kind of perspective that I was lacking in my life.*

Every day during my meditation sessions I repeated to myself: *I am here for a reason, there are synchronicities at work in my life that are beyond coincidence. I deserve everything I want. I deserve wellness, and I am a deeply happy, healthy, nurtured, and loving human being at my core.*

SAD

My Brahman was not God-realization, but self-realization, and it was very real. I, along with many other people, suffer from a condition that's been termed seasonal affective disorder (SAD). Folks with SAD become severely depressed during winter months without any apparent cause. Medicine now recognizes that light sensitivity may have a lot to do with the pineal gland, or the "third eye," which is a small, oval endocrine gland within the vertebrate brain that responds to changes in sunlight. Nearly all vertebrate species, except the hagfish—an eel-shaped, slime-producing marine fish that is thought to be the most primitive of vertebrates (and looks like something out of a lucid nightmare)—possess a pineal gland.

For me, SAD had more to do with being stuck indoors for long hours. It affected everything from the endless hours in my small apartment helplessly watching the snow climb up my windows, to the two hours spent digging my car out of the snow before work. Winter had given me acute frostbite (waiting over an hour for a bus during my fieldwork term in Boston), had forced me to cancel rent-paying jobs, and was overall super unproductive for my life. I spent my winter days looking forward to long naps, had fallen into more snowbanks than I could count, had lost feeling in my toes on so very many long walks to class, and had experienced a cold that immediately made its way to my bones and wouldn't leave. Rainy days would make me burst out crying for no apparent reason and I felt hopeless and anxious all the time. My bones ached at the slightest change in temperature. I'd feel great during meditations, then open my curtains to a gray day and feel sunken all over again.

My lack of motivation and the short days that come with winter in New England were the least of my worries. On top of just being very down about things never going as planned with crappy weather, it was equally depressing to have random bouts of sadness I couldn't explain, emotional outbursts, and seemingly no life resilience. I just couldn't ever wait for winter to be *over*.

I came off my medication in March 2011. With a bitter chill still in the air and spring just on the horizon, next year's winter was absolutely sickening for me to even think about. What struck me first was that SAD was a natural body response to an environment that I had spent every day in for twenty-four years. It was not a "disorder" or something that required medication for me, but *it was very real*, and it did require a huge step. I needed to move.

About a month after I came off my medication, I started seriously thinking about moving. And I finally had to think outside of the box. Anytime I had moved from New York, whether it was going to Bennington College in Vermont or going to Boston between December and February for that frostbite-inducing fieldwork term, I had never made a move based on sunshine or wellness. I had always stayed in my comfort zone or moved for someone else.

So, my next move was easy: to find some place with sunshine that allowed me to keep fulfilling my destiny of optimum mental and physical health, even if I was super far away. And to do it for me.

Follow Your Heart

I researched places to live with a new, inspired attitude. I left myself completely open to anywhere, and Google Earthed myself throughout most of the country. Oregon, Colorado, Texas, Florida, Arizona, and New Mexico were all on my map. But one place kept calling out to me.

California.

I had only been to California once, maybe a year or so before. I'd taken a random trip to San Francisco, much to the dismay of my possessive boyfriend. While there I had wandered around gawking at palm trees, explored the redwoods, hiked Muir Woods, brunched on the bay, experienced a bone-chilling cold I couldn't explain, smoked a lot of medical marijuana to combat my pain, and batted off advances from the person I stayed with for four days. I left thinking, *This has got to be the New York of California. I should have stayed home.*

Still, I had a feeling that Southern California held a different appeal than what I had experienced in northern San Francisco. So while I didn't have any model to go by—my entire family, as well as all of my oldest friends, were in *and always had been* in New York—I decided to *just look.* I researched a little bit, and asked Henry for advice, because he had lived in California before. He expressed a sincere desire to move with me, and suggested Los Angeles, specifically North Hollywood. He said North Hollywood was more suburban than Hollywood or Downtown Los Angeles, and was great for people who just moved or were just starting out.

Synchronicity

It was late June 2011 and I was apartment hunting on Craigslist for places in Hollywood. Sipping green juice, I emailed exactly two people inquiring about their "For Rent" places. One was a studio apartment in North Hollywood and the other was a smaller studio apartment closer to Culver City. I told them I was interested, lived in NYC currently, sent a photo of myself along with my phone number and email address. I didn't really expect a reply.

Shortly after, I got one. Within a day or two, the North Hollywood apartment emailed back. *Hi there,* she wrote. *My name is Raca. What a coincidence! I am moving back to New York and would love to talk to you about the apartment.* We set up a time to call one another and I was happy, but a little apprehensive. I wasn't exactly committed to moving to some place I had never seen before.

A few minutes before our scheduled time to call, I got a text from Raca. *I thought I recognized you!* it said. *We grew up together!*

I read it in confusion.

Where? I texted back. I had never seen a picture of this person and I was certain I didn't ever grow up with anyone who had moved to California.

Well, we didn't, she explained. *Oh man! I was almost positive but now I'm certain. Your cousin is my best friend. We did dance together growing up. I know you! I am moving back to New York to pursue dance again, and your cousin Amory is one of the first people I will be seeing! What a coincidence!*

I read the text from Raca over and over and over again. My heart raced with excitement and disbelief. I broke into a huge smile. My cousins were like my sisters growing up. Amory and Jade, both close to me in age, were avid dancers since they were toddlers until college. I had gone to many of their practices, recitals, rehearsals, and shows, and attended a lot of birthday parties with their friends.

When Raca and I finally spoke on the phone, we both acknowledged how absolutely incredible it was that at the time I would be looking for an apartment after almost twenty-five years in New York, Raca's would be up for rent! We acknowledged how amazing it was that I was only really just *thinking* about moving, and so far had only been compelled to contact two people after looking for days, and Raca was one of them. We laughed at how beautiful it was that she was moving *back* to the same place I was moving *from,* and that my family had indeed had a huge hand in her decision. Talk about synchronicity!

Raca pep-talked me about moving across the country, assured me about the safe neighborhood she lived in, and raved about the weather. She even encouraged my move, and told me it was always nice to have a fresh start. This girl I had actually—unbeknownst to me—grown up with assured me I'd make a lot of friends just by having an open mind. She was only moving back to New York because the dance scene was better. Things were different in California, she explained. People were, well, *nicer*.

"If you decide to do it," she said, "it'll be so easy. I'll even leave you my furniture. And your family will feel totally safe. I'll assure them it's a great neighborhood, and *it really is*. I can talk to anyone you want about it. I can even try to get the landlord here to lower the rent I posted."

It did seem a little too good to be true that I could really approach my family about moving by saying I was taking my cousin's best friend's apartment in California. Not that I needed my family's approval to move, but damn, it would be helpful to have some support, since I was scared about it myself. I knew it would significantly soften the blow if I was changing my life and heading to a safe environment.

When I really decided to do it, I didn't turn back. I sent my rent deposit a good two months before I moved, just to secure the place. This was really frightening for me, and I spent quite a few nights at home crying about the idea of leaving everything and everyone I knew for . . . what? What was supposed to be out there for me again?

Travel. A wellness-centered new lifestyle. A change. An adventure. Right, but was it really worth finding someone else to move into my apartment, giving up everything I'd known, packing all of my stuff, and moving over three thousand miles to some place I'd *never actually even seen* before? Could I really move to a city I had never been to in my life? With no guarantee of getting a job, a résumé that was corporate and scientific at best (neither types of jobs I wanted anyway), no friends, and absolutely no guarantee of happiness at all?

Personal Power

For some reason, I was all about it. I knew that, if nothing else, what I had done forever *wasn't working*. No matter where I turned, I was still miserable, no matter whom I spoke to, no one was really trying to find their own happiness or peace, and no matter what I did, a part of me really just couldn't be happy where I was. I knew I had to *become the change* to *see* any change in my life.

Also, adventure sounded really fun.

I let my boss know of my plans to move, helped him hire my replacement, and without an ounce of remorse or regret, I left my laboratory job analyzing asbestos samples on July 1. I was a little at odds about what to do, so I applied for a few acting jobs. It had been a week since I applied to the last one, and I had only been thinking of it sporadically. Since I hadn't heard anything, I just let it simmer.

I was still getting very sick, but I had enough saved up that I wasn't worried about money quite yet. This gave me the first opportunity in my whole life to focus on getting well. I gave everything up to my Personal Power.

Getting Well

Not only was my family happy for me when I told them I was moving, they were actually incredibly supportive. Dad, I swear, beamed when I told him. Although he was apprehensive about his little girl moving so far, I knew he was proud of me for making such a big decision for myself.

Leave it to two Irish immigrants to be more than supportive about me moving three thousand miles away to pursue my dreams.

Well, we also had a slight advantage: Dad had worked for the airlines since the year he moved here, at eighteen years old. This meant that traveling to and from New York and Los Angeles might not be a problem, depending on the circumstance.

My grandparents told me that if I felt the need to move, to do it. We had very reassuring talks about my decision. I often traveled there for late-night tea with Grandma to talk out my feelings.

The most reassuring part to me was that it was *my* decision. No one had pressured me to move to California, or anywhere for that matter. I already lived somewhere, I had already held a job, I had already started growing roots somewhere. It was actually a pretty bad time to have come off all my medication, realize my true potential, and move across the country, because my life was finally secure and comfortable.

After considering many options, I decided that getting in a car and driving was the best one. A road trip would allow me to explore more places, learn more things, encounter more people, and have many more adventures. I felt like it was Now, or Never.

Unlike many of my so-called friends at the time, who questioned every step I took along the way, my family actually made me feel very comfortable about moving to LA, and they were especially reassured when I told them I was moving into my cousin's best friend's apartment. They agreed with me that the kind of synchronicity that had made such a large plan into a tangible reality *doesn't just happen.*

Once I had my family's encouragement, things started falling into place rapidly. Some of those acting jobs I had applied for weeks ago came rolling in.

First, I got a random phone call from a casting director. She said she had a featured part for me in a new movie by an Academy Award–winning director, and some of my favorite actors and actresses were the stars. She asked if I could make it to a fitting that week. *Could I?* I jumped around my room screaming of happiness, my heart bursting at the seams. I kissed Raelie a hundred times.

I signed onto the project without hesitation.

Working for Yourself

I had modeled briefly at the age of eighteen during my summers home from college, and was on a fast track to the top, with a magazine cover, a major ad, and a full-page fashion spread under my belt in the first few months. But this kind of modeling was a full-time gig—the kind where your other job needs to "understand" that you have castings all day long, and you have to drop out of school or be privately tutored. Education always held a higher appeal for me, so I'd given modeling up completely.

I had a feeling that I could do it again, and was itching to do artistic, creative projects. I put an ad on a popular model/photographer website and hoped for the best.

I got a lot of great responses and started working that same week. It was through doing creative modeling projects again that I met some of the most influential and incredible people I have ever known and reawakened a career I had all but abandoned a whopping five years before. I fell right back into it the first day as if I had never stopped, and actually found myself doing better, acting more confident, becoming more talkative, friendly, and playing muse to others. I only did a handful of small gigs, but fate provided the exact right relationships. I was tapped in.

You need to be a good boss to work for yourself. This was the first time other people started to perk up and notice that I was, in essence, working for myself at twenty-four years old. I had an easier time paying the bills working for myself than I ever had when I worked a nine-to-five (always an 8:00 a.m. to possibly 8:00 a.m. the next day for me, but y'know). I set my modeling fee at almost ten times higher an hour than what I had made at my last place of employment, and was very selective about whom I worked with. I prepped myself for acting in my first feature film.

Acting

It was just a day or two after getting the call about the feature film that I got another call. It was from the producer of a major news network TV show. They were doing a story, they said, on sugar daddies. Was I familiar with this concept?

In all honesty, I was not. They explained sugar daddies to me: older men who often pay college-aged girls that they find on the Internet for their company. This honestly didn't sound like the worst thing in the world to me, but it wasn't necessarily the most appealing thing either. However, the network was willing to hire me to do an undercover story about sugar daddies. They assured me that I'd have an Emmy Award–winning mentor for this piece, and I'd be taking down some real sleazebags. I would be the bait, trying to trick guys into admitting that they would be giving me an allowance to sleep with them. I needed to get these men to say exactly what they wanted, and—most importantly—that they were willing to pay for it. The network would need my permission, they said, to use my photograph and a fake name of my choosing to lure these men on websites. Then I would meet the guys on a date or during lunch while they filmed. A reporter would come out once the date was over and "confront" the men, much like *To Catch a Predator.*

I was very hesitant about this. It sounded shady as hell and possibly dangerous. Not only would it require acting skills *I wasn't sure that I had*, it felt super manipulative. *These guys were probably lonely*, I thought, *and I think everyone should be able to make money however they want to.*

However, things all changed once they talked to me about my real goal: making sure girls didn't get hurt. Some of these girls, the network told me, had talked to them about being completely manipulated in their sugar daddy relationships. That was their real story, and that really changed my mind.

Also, my day rate for this job would be exactly enough to make my move to California incredible. I wouldn't have to worry about rent for a few months once I moved.

I told them I'd do it. It was only August and I wouldn't be filming the feature until October. Henry and I had planned to leave for California the day after I filmed the feature: Wednesday, October 19.

I spent September 1, 2011, my twenty-fifth birthday, sick as a dog. Henry and I went to Pure Food and Wine, a raw-food restaurant in New York City, and all I could talk about was how sick I was and how excited I was to not be in New York anymore. I had half a cocktail and spent the entire night over the toilet bowl. Oops.

The undercover network news job was just as shady and strange as I thought it was going to be, but it did do two things.

First, it rapidly improved my skills. Like whoa. Like, damn. I had forced myself into a situation where failure was not an option. The cell phone I had with me during these "dates" was one that the network had given me, and the famous reporter—who *was* becoming a mentor to me—was sending texts to me with instructions. My purse was a camera. They also hired people who were filming with hidden cameras in plain clothes around me. It was a sting, and I was the bait.

Some of these guys never showed up to the dates the network had set up, but a lot of them actually *did*. I talked to some very powerful people connected to companies I'd rather not name, but most of them were former business moguls or the heads of very large corporations. And they all had a sob story. One man told me his wife had cancer for ten years and he had been taking care of her five children from another marriage the entire time. He was exhausted, he said, and just wanted some company.

I had to convince these strangers to open up to me, and I did it expertly. A few of the guys did get confronted about offering to pay me for sex or company, and they were deeply embarrassed. My mentor was often cheering me on and giving me big hugs afterward, calling me incredibly brave. I could feel my acting skills improving each and every day. I was psyched.

Second, it validated everything. Did I really just get a "dream job" that might pay for absolutely all of my expenses, just weeks after quitting my "real" job? Was I really that much closer to what I wanted? I was making connections, I was improving rapidly at my craft, I was surrounded by amazing mentors. It validated absolutely everything that I was working on. It made me so, so happy that I had made the decision and quit my lab job just two months ago! I was making more in a day at this new job than what I was making in a week at my old job. Was this my new life?

Hope

It was around this time that Dad came down with very strange symptoms. It took a lot of convincing, but we finally got him to see a doctor. He was quickly diagnosed with stage IV cancer. It was a type of renal cell carcinoma that had popped up in his kidney. He didn't have much of a chance, the oncologist said, unless they took his kidney out. Even then, the doctor gave him only six months to live. We were all devastated.

At least once they took the mass out, they could test it, find out what it was, and give him the right treatment. After the initial shock wore off, my family was actually very hopeful. A close relative had been in remission from a rare spinal cancer for thirteen years, citing herbs, yoga, and lifestyle change for his recovery. Dad had survived worse—even once coming down with a mysterious infection that left him right at death's door before he miraculously made an overnight comeback with no drugs at all.

I was apprehensive about moving to California immediately upon hearing about the surgery. Everything in me wanted to stay, to be with him as much as I could. I wanted to do every-thing in my power to help him, and I wanted to make him proud of me in the short time we might have left together. The idea that he might only be around for *six more months* was daunting and terrifying.

I realized that the best medicine I could give him would be to live my life. I was determined to be happy, to have a beau-tiful life I could share with my family, and to be stable enough to care for Dad if he needed it. I wanted to show by example. This was a radical thought for me, and it swelled me with pride and hope.

Making the Commitment

I had made the commitment to moving. My grandparents were actually the ones who encouraged me to move to California *the most,* even after Dad's diagnosis. There was nothing I could do from home, they said, even if I stayed. I knew they were right. I also knew I'd be home for Thanksgiving, Christmas, New Year's, and perhaps I could find some excuses to come back other times during the year.

I was successfully making a chance for myself to succeed, despite my own health issues, despite my family's, and despite whatever may happen. My mind was focused on finding healthy coping mechanisms instead of running all the time. And moving was not running; it was very much doing the opposite of what my heart was telling me to do—stay with my father, my grandfather, my adoptive dad, through his struggles, illness, surgeries, and challenges. But I had committed to move, and my soul was fully on board.

Failure was no longer an option for me. This was also a totally radical thought and created an amazing shift in my life. I was certain that I could do more to help him if I moved than if I stayed home.

My days with the network were winding down, and I was taking odd modeling jobs, working on my wellness, and counting down the days to the feature film and the road trip.

The First Feature

On October 18, 2011, I did my featured part in my first major movie, which included a scene with a famous movie star. It ended up getting cut from the final edit of the movie, but it served its purpose tremendously: it was my first taste of feature films and professional acting, and I was totally hooked. Not to mention the fact that the celebrity I had filmed a scene with started following me on Twitter and tweeted at me immediately after the shoot! How cool!

I had missed acting, even if only for a few moments a day. Although most of the day on set for the movie had been spent in a back room waiting to get called, I learned that this was actually a very normal part of the business, and those few hours I was in front of the camera were totally magical to me.

My day on set was a whirlwind, which ultimately led to great revelations of my own. I met and worked with everyone, including the star and the Academy Award–winning director, and it all felt totally *normal*. The star of the movie was the most professional man I have had the pleasure of working with. We filmed on a busy New York City street corner in front of a Halloween shop—I think it was on 42nd Street, or maybe a block or two over from the busy Seventh Avenue intersection. After a few minutes, there was a throng of paparazzi in the street and across the sidewalk taking photos. He introduced himself as if he wasn't *the entire reason* they were there, shook everyone's hand, including strange tourists, signed autographs, and politely asked if everyone would go across the street to take photos. Everyone obliged.

It was the nicest thing I had seen anyone do in business *period*, and it was definitely the nicest thing I've ever even heard of a celebrity doing, never mind seen one do in person. *Why don't gossip columns write about this stuff?* I thought. It gave me a huge personal goal about how to act in general. My entire body exploded with possibility. I wanted to be the nicest, most professional, respectful, humble person I knew. *Period.*

That one, single, beautiful day on set was a complete game changer. Seeing the star of the film treating his fans with such respect and humility was the most inspiring thing I had ever seen. My meditation visualizations started to become stronger immediately, because almost everything I had already visualized was becoming real. I looked forward to my meditations, instead of dreading them like I had done in the beginning. I knew that my mind held all the secret solutions to all the things I wanted. I couldn't wait to get home and meditate.

Suddenly meditation not only felt like a secret relaxation technique that no one else knew about, but it also absolutely helped me visualize my life *as I would have liked it to be.* I was becoming better, stronger, and more healthy and motivated by the day. I often had to interrupt my meditations to write down my ideas, and *even that* didn't bother me. In fact, it reminded me of when I used to write down all of my thoughts as a kid. Except this time, I wasn't jotting things down because I woke up in the middle of the night due to insomnia, my emotions, or my tears. I was getting everything done early during the day, and sleeping soundly at night.

I had a feeling that my decision to move to Los Angeles, Home of the Feature Film, "the land of fruits and nuts" (as Dad would say), had been a good one. Even though I had made this commitment, actually packing all my stuff was very emotional for me. I cried almost every day. I wrote a ton of journal entries about how I felt, pouring my heart out into barely tangible words every night.

Fortunately, I had found a relative to move into my New York apartment, so I felt better about leaving the place. I knew I'd be able to visit whenever I wanted to.

In just the past nine months, I had done everything from going to an ex's funeral, breaking up with a boyfriend of three years, and trying to kill myself, to coming off all my medication, committing to changing myself, deciding to move, and dealing with my dad's cancer diagnosis—regardless of how it ended. Nine months. Wow. And I was the most fired-up and excited about life that I'd been . . . *ever.* Even though every single event could have been seen as the most depressing and hardest thing I had faced yet, I didn't want to be a victim to my circumstances anymore. This was another true breakthrough that started to make *The Dream* so real.

CREATING MOMENTUM

I had immediately begun to create momentum in my life, which is one of the most powerful steps in creating the life you desire. Keep in mind, I was still very sick, a little discouraged, and totally apprehensive because I had *never really changed anything in my life before. I had no idea where to start.* But I took steps to create momentum and propel my life forward anyway. Taking the necessary steps to force your life into motion will work for you no matter where you are at on your journey.

DECIDE YOURSELF

Decisions both large and small had pushed me to decide what I was worth, and to whom. They forced me to step back and ask, "Who am I?" which motivated even more behaviors that established who I was. We are all a work in progress, and that means that at every moment, we're *choosing* to be who we are. Even little decisions, like knowing how gently to brush our hair, deciding what food to eat to fuel us, or treating ourselves like who we always wanted to be, all add up to our perspective of ourselves, which we then confirm to ourselves after making our new decisions. Take a moment to evaluate where you are in your life and what you are currently doing with it. How many of those decisions were yours and how many of those were made for you?

MOTIVATE YOURSELF

I needed to give myself a reason to *take action immediately.* Whether it was getting a job that very day that forced me to tune up on my acting skills, telling my family I was moving to confirm the move for myself, or seeking support from friends, these were all ways I was giving myself *no other option* but to change my life and do something different. Motivation comes in all kinds of different forms, and only you know what's actually going to force you to take action.

The best way to motivate yourself is to share your dreams with friends or family members who will hold you to your dreams and encourage you to accomplish them. This way, you will not only have the support of your loved ones through all of your endeavors, but you will also be forced to live up to your standards constantly.

You're either getting better or worse. You're either going forward or backward. In life, there is no standing still. You owe it to yourself to give *You* no other choice but to constantly improve.

INTERRUPT YOURSELF

I had to *interrupt old life patterns* in order to establish new ones. Every time I felt a panic attack coming on, for example, instead of giving into it or reaching for a drug, I would stop to realize what was happening and start my favorite breathing exercise, or go somewhere to be alone and calm down. Or I'd write, or read a book that I knew would comfort me.

Soon, *every feeling of panic turned into a moment of excitement where I could focus and change everything for the better.* Instead of giving into old patterns like self-harm and self-abuse, I did loving things, like taking out my frustrations in music and writing, creating healthy, vibrant meals, and working on my relationships with other people. I found a replacement for old behaviors, and was therefore getting rid of old neural pathways, and changing them into better, new neural pathways as I went along.

CONDITION YOURSELF

I needed to condition myself by creating constant and long-term change. I knew that this would only really happen with time, but that each and every moment of every day needed to be dedicated to self-realization, wellness, and finding my own form of peace. I needed to develop my own coping mechanisms so that I could face my life—no matter what happened—without relying on anyone else or having a breakdown. I wanted to be capable of making myself well even when I was sad, and I wanted to be capable of dealing with Dad's diagnosis, or perhaps, as I feared, even death, the best way I could without checking myself into a mental institution, without going back on medication, and without relying on other people. I wanted to be able to do it naturally, effectively, long-term, and *unconditionally.*

Classical conditioning is actually a Pavlovian concept. The guy who rang a bell every time he brought a dog its food, then watched it salivate after he rang a bell but produced no food? That's your guy. But it works for humans really well too. We use it everywhere.

Conditioning is the basic concept for commercials—why a company plays a certain commercial over and over instead of, say, making five different commercials and rotating them. We use it every day. We just do it unconsciously. Conditioning is behavior modification. And we've figured out approximately how long it takes for a human to turn a habit into a different habit, how long it takes to develop a new personality trait, a new muscle, or a new you.

It takes twenty-one days. I know this not only because I've read it in practically every self-help book there is, but because I've practiced it. And it works.

It took me around three weeks to change my palate from registering kale as totally tasteless to really feeling like it was the best thing I had ever eaten. It took me about a month to go from devouring a pint of ice cream to craving pomegranate seeds. It took me approximately a month of sobriety to make me realize I couldn't take a pill to change a thought.

When you condition yourself—every moment, every day—to become the person you want to be, to smile in the face of fear, to say no when your body and everything you've let say YES for years tries to scream YES, you'll find a different kind of happiness. The happiness that comes with control. Real control. The kind of control where you can step back, look clearly at things, and think, *I really understand myself today.*

"I Can't!"

By the time I set out on the road trip, I was completely ready to do everything but one thing: I wasn't ready to leave Raelie behind.

If you let them, dogs can be as close to you as a child, and they act like family members right off the bat. This felt a lot like leaving my little girl behind.

Many people get stuck right here. Despite leaving my job, despite giving my deposit, despite telling everyone, despite packing and finding someone else to move into my place, I still could have changed my mind. The thoughts of "I can't!" are what trap us in our limiting mentalities and subsequent limiting behaviors and their subsequent limiting actions. Things as simple as being told we're unworthy, having acne or a discouraging partner, or the idea that we can't leave someone who loves us keep us stuck and suffocated in the same small spaces we've always been hiding in for comfort. We say *we can't* because we're afraid that *we can*.

The Course by Marianne Williamson explains, "The ego is totally confused, and totally confusing." You can say that again! My ego was all over the place. One minute I was a self-assured "former" scientist with an incredible résumé behind me and a great future in front of me. Next, I was a confused little girl who stood to lose everything: my family, my friends, my comfort zone, my dog.

Accessing our Personal Power is the solution to "I can't" and its limiting mentalities. Until I could find a way to get her to California, Raelie was to stay in New York, the place I was so desperate to escape. I turned the apartment over to a relative, who promised to care for Raelie as her own.

With this last detail in place, I had absolutely no excuses left to make me anxious about the road trip. I was ready.

CHAPTER SIX

HOW TO CREATE LASTING CHANGE

"Paradise is not found in a place. It's a state of consciousness."
—Sri Chinmoy (1931–2007), Spiritual Teacher, Meditation Guru, Prolific Renaissance Man, Badass New Yorker

I had a ton of energy and inspiration, and was making big plans. I started drawing, painting, and writing again for the first time in many, many years. I was pleasantly surprised to find that I could still do these things as if I had never skipped a beat. These artistic forms of expression had been my favorite activities and therapies as a kid, yet somehow I'd forgotten about how integral they were to my happiness, my identity, and my true being.

Most importantly, I started making my own music again. I was not afraid to go to a studio and jam out with strangers, sing in the shower, sing in front of my family, or sing my heart out at a microphone. I loved making up words as they came lucidly to my head. I had actually never improvised my lyrics or sung for my family, or done most of these things openly before, but I became more and more pumped up on the idea of doing that with an audience in front of me. I sang in the kitchen, at the grocery store, in front of strangers. I harmonized with every song that I heard. I was tired of closing my life to the outside world, and tired of always being afraid of what other people thought of me. I was very set on developing a whole new attitude on life. I was eager to do more things I enjoyed, embrace new coping mechanisms that were starting to mold my life into something I sort of recognized and was proud of.

The only time these new coping methods I'd developed didn't work was, again, when I didn't believe in them. On days where I felt impossibly sick, or on days I felt like I "deserved" to feel sad, I had absolutely no power to feel better. I realized, eventually, that I had *designed it this way*.

Why Would We Make Ourselves Sick?

I designed it this way because I was scared. I was scared of what would happen if I stayed sick, and the longer I was sick, the more scared I would become about *what I'd have to do with my life if and when I got better*. I knew that the sorts of jobs that I had in the past had contributed *immensely and undeniably* to my illness. It felt like a huge roadblock on the path to complete wellness.

This kind of escapism or excuse is fairly common, but at the time, for me it was an especially frightening thought. The justification of "This is all I know. How can I possibly change? How could I do something else?" haunted me, even as I embraced new changes and ideas about who I was. This question haunts each one of us in our own way at some point or another. It is often hard for us to picture another way of life, and the *longer we stay in a situation, the more difficult it becomes to picture our lives differently*. Chronic pain, chronic illness, or relationships gone bad are some of the many, many things that keep us from the daily, blissful, pure happiness that we all truly deserve. *If we see pain, there is pain*.

Miracles are not reserved for saints alone. We all have the ability to create miracles in our lives, including ridding our bodies of pain, aches, grief, and sadness. All of us have the ability to cure ourselves, each and every day. I didn't believe this then, even though I *thought* I knew deeply about psychosomatics at the time.

Psychosomatics refers to the intimate relationships between your thoughts and the way your body behaves. Since the time of Hippocrates—medical guru of ancient Greece—doctors have been puzzled by how patients could be cured (often of terminal illness!) with absolutely no medical intervention. Anyone and *anything* can inflict pain upon us, but it is up to us alone to find a way to deal with it. We *all* have the capacity to create beliefs around events that make those events empowering. Great tragedies, death, chronic illness, cancer, abuse, or stressors like day-to-day chores, work, or a bad breakup can be recognized as meaningful things with the capacity to shape us positively.

I once told myself again and again, "I just can't," when a voice whispered to me, "Of course you can!" It was That Voice—the one that knew the right thing to do, and did it. To anyone who feels defeated by life or trapped by illness, circumstance, or a haunting memory, listen to the voice that again and again says, "Of course you can." It may be whispering now, but you need to let it have its time to speak up. It has valuable things to say. Let that voice become louder and louder. Let it encourage you to defy all of your odds, instead of entrapping yourself in and being defined by them.

I knew I would suffer from chronic illness and melancholy forever if I went back to "old habits" like giving in to anxiety, breathing wrong from panic, taking prescription medication when I was stressed, or resorting to my worst drug: escaping into other people, drama, and problems. Worry and stress both perpetuate disease and anxiety. They are poisonous to carry around with us!

Many of us make ourselves sick because it's easier to have an excuse. We'd like to think that our emotions aren't in our control, that our destiny is in the hands of fate or is reliant on someone else, or that our future is doomed to turn out in a particular way because of a diagnosis, disease, or our past.

"Anything you're good at contributes to happiness."
—Bertrand Russell (1872–1970),
British Philosopher, Writer, Social Critic, Historian

Stop Worrying & Start Living

The first step in changing these excuses is to realize that your emotions are completely in your control, and that you alone are the one choosing to give in to any negative emotions that may lead you straight to negative actions. I had always wondered why I couldn't stop myself during panic attacks, but I finally realized it was because *I had never done so before*. I had never conditioned myself to do anything *any* differently than what I had always done, which was give into the fear and anxiety!

I was the only person responsible for the life I had because *only I had created it*. Yes, other people had been there. Other people had influenced it. Yes, other people had even *convinced me that they ruled it*. Yes, I often felt completely helpless to my circumstances, my health, my bank account, and my surrounding company. But I realized that I had brought all of those things *on myself and into my whole life*. I had allowed other people to be there, to influence how I felt, and to provoke a reaction in me. Only I had allowed myself to panic or stress out. Most importantly, only I had spent all the money I had made. No one had robbed me.

The idea that "no one taught me how to manage my money" or "no one taught me how to love" got thrown right out of my mentality. I recognized them for what they were: Excuses, with a capital E. I realized that a wealth of knowledge—millions of books, hours and hours of free lectures—existed out there, and if I accessed it, I could really change my life.

I also realized that I had never *thought* highly of myself, never *treated* myself well. This uninspired view of myself had been based on how other people had treated me, and became even more ingrained in my mind the day a doctor told me that I was mentally ill and that I would have to take a drug for the rest of my life to function normally.

This manifested as preconceived notions of who *I thought* I was based on my family, my history, my upbringing, the pharmaceutical drugs I was taking . . . Not only were the drugs themselves having an effect, the idea that *I needed the drugs was also having an effect*—doubling the crippling blow to my self-worth.

Then I ironically lived that notion based on my views—which were also based on other people's views—and had confirmed it over and over and over for myself. I realized that I had spent years denying myself things I truly felt that I deserved, not making art I wanted to make, not talking to people I wanted to talk to, not pursuing the career that I wanted to have, all because of this belief that I didn't deserve it. This now seemed totally crazy to me.

Don't get me wrong: I'd had this epiphany in small doses before. I had tried a lot of tactics in the past to change this half-realization, but I always found myself crawling at a snail's pace in my personal growth. Always trying to catch up to a flimsy glimpse of who I felt I should be. I'd look at other people's lives and careers with scathing, envious resentment. "Why isn't that me?" I'd ask, sipping on a cocktail with one hand and searching for the bottle of Lamictal with the other.

I even tried to bully myself into changing, as we often do. I'd ruined relationships, failed tests, lost apartments, put myself in an abusive partnership, and otherwise tried changing my habits by giving myself "no other choice." I had no other choice, all right. But instead of changing my life for the better, I ended up strung out on prescribed drugs, homeless, friendless, living in my car, on welfare, and in violent and unhealthy relationships all by my early twenties. In the past I had hit "rock bottom," and I let someone else help me get back up.

I taught myself how to change by studying the lives of my role models. I had a lot of time when I was lying sick in bed to reflect on my life choices, and a lot of them had been doozies. However, when I looked back now, something was definitely different. Instead of seeing myself as an awful person capable of only terrible things, I saw myself as a vulnerable human being who was always making the choice she felt was best at the time. I was totally understanding of myself as a fallible human being who hadn't been anywhere close to perfect, but I still had a chance. Yes, I had made many mistakes. But they were mistakes I never wanted to make again. *If I can leave that person in the past,* I thought, *I'll be okay.*

I spent a great deal of time listening to the same Tony Robbins tapes that I had enjoyed as a kid. I read a ton of autobiographies, including Gandhi's, Amelia Earhart's, Richard Branson's, Lucille Ball's, Dolly Parton's, Ethel Merman's, and Benjamin Franklin's. Any new idea I wanted to learn, I did so by finding a role model and looking into how they lived, how they thought, and what they did that made them different than everyone else.

How to Create Lasting Change

So, what had changed? Nothing around me, that was for sure. The economy, my family, my job, my friends, my neighborhood, my co-workers, my past, everything I had been through, all stayed pretty much exactly the same. However, the most important thing that could have changed, had changed. *I* had changed. Furthermore, I was *committed* to that change; it wasn't just a belief, or a thought, or a wish. I knew in my heart what I was capable of, who I wanted to become, where I wanted to live, and what I wanted my life to look like. I believed in this even when other people didn't believe in it, didn't approve of it, or didn't understand it. I believed in it so strongly that I no longer required anyone else's approval. This had compelled me to act accordingly, to live every single moment toward becoming that person.

This is exactly what prevents us from getting into limiting life patterns and feelings of being "stuck." I was accessing my Personal Power which truly comes when you stop pointing the finger, even at yourself. This isn't about blaming yourself. This is about *becoming* yourself.

Ask Triggering Questions

Asking questions that trigger positive action is the only way to create lasting change in your life, your career, your bank account, your relationships, or whatever you're trying to gain control over. When we ask ourselves questions like, "What would happen if I don't change?" we're linking our feelings of pain to negative patterns of behavior.

I was determined to find a solution to my problems, because I knew that a life following practically the same path as my good friend (whose solution had been to take her own life) was *not* where I wanted to go. The scars I had from my own brush with death changed from an embarrassment to a daily reminder of a place I never wanted to see again. Instead of being something I cringed at, my scars seemed more like a tattoo. A reminder of another time and place in my life. A choice I had made. They were also a blaring sign that clearly read: **NEVER DO THIS AGAIN!**

Once I looked my fears straight in the face, I realized how much they had been controlling me, and it wasn't long before I realized something else remarkable: they *weren't even real.* They were just *beliefs* I had carried with me about things, and I could change them at any moment, *in a moment.*

Create Change in a Moment

True freedom was the ability to face my fears and tell them to go fuck themselves. Fears are funny little beliefs we have that trigger chemical reactions in us. They usually mean different things for different people. The same thing that scares someone to death, like jumping out of a plane, is a sport that someone like Guinness World Record holder Don Kellner has done over forty-two thousand times since 1961, purely for fun!

Here are important steps to help you in your quest to truly tackle your fears for good and find true freedom. Reference them when you are getting frustrated in your personal growth. Most importantly, practice them! Practicing new behaviors is the only way to permanently change your brain chemistry, and ultimately, your actions, your personality, and your life.

Stop Giving a Crap What Others Think

Every single journal entry I wrote before the age of twenty-four featured the same theme over and over: they always referenced someone else. "Spent the day with Joe at the park . . ." "Katie and I hung out at her house and drank green tea . . ." "Hung out with Paul and Zack today . . ." Page after page focused on other people.

I used to be ruled by my relationships: my relationships to people, drugs, teachers, strangers, food, family, my significant others. It had taken years, but I was finally no longer willing to entertain anyone else's thoughts of me or what I should be doing with my life or my time.

Realize Other People Are Wrong

Okay, okay. They're not *always* wrong. And I certainly didn't dismiss other people's opinions or advice. In fact, for the first time in my life, this is when *I actually truly heard them.* I saw myself listening for the first time ever. I took advice, I considered things people told me about myself without getting insulted or defensive. I improved on my behaviors, I got nicer in my speech, and I adopted new words and mannerisms to express myself. However, I also saw other people's opinions for exactly what they were: *their own* beliefs, based on *their own* life experience, *and they were just as fallible as I was.*

People are subject to human error. And that's okay! (It just means they're not robots.) It's important to acknowledge that human error shows up in all kinds of ways. I just stopped getting offended and defensive about how other people thought I should live. I simply listened.

Realize Other People's Beliefs Change

If other people were just as fallible as I was, that meant that just like my opinions, their opinions could change. They often had. First of all, as far as I was concerned, everyone else had been *dead wrong* about what I was capable of for as long as I could remember. I had heard I "couldn't do everything" and that I had to start "being realistic" my entire life. I was always discouraged from doing things "my way." Even at my progressive college, my four mentors (the classic average was one—two at most) sat me down to advise me to "concentrate on acting."

I asked them all, *Why?*

When I finally started to realize that I could do whatever I put my mind to *regardless of anyone else's opinions*, and that "being realistic" was the surest way to dissolve my dreams for another five years, I started to take other people's opinions with a grain of salt. They had their place if they were positive, but other than that I wasn't going to stand around and be told *what I could not do*.

Finding this conviction is the difference between getting the job during the interview and losing it to the next person. It's the difference between continuing your business in its current direction and knowing when you need to change course. It's the difference between creating a life of stability and always feeling like you're a few steps behind.

Ironically, the second I started to accomplish my goals, other people's opinions about what I was capable of changed immediately. Suddenly it was expected that everything I did was wildly successful and fun, because that was the image I had created by living my life that way. This helped me evaluate what *I really could do* and inspired me to become more and more a person that former naysayers now believed in.

Once you have a foundation for who you want to be, and you begin to accomplish those goals, you are setting the stage for other people's opinions of you. Recognize that other people are also human, beautiful, fallible, funny, fucked up, and everything in between. More importantly *what other people say does not determine who you are*. This is crucial to lasting change.

Leave the Judgments at the Door

Take the time to pause before you judge someone—at least out loud. You can't take your words back. When we pause, we can even start to rephrase our thoughts about a certain someone or even about the situation itself. When we step back from judgment, we can truly begin to reevaluate what place it has in our lives. We begin to get control of our own mind.

In order to stop being ruled by my relationships immediately, I made it simple for myself: if I had a judgment, question, or theory about someone else's life choices, I just *asked them about it.* I noticed (in pretty short order) that many people got very defensive when I asked them about their lives or plans or current situations, and that was because I was, in essence, *being judgmental.* But a lot of people opened up to me. And after a few days of this I realized how silly (and hypocritical) it was of me to have judgments about anyone else at all, and how much time it had taken away from my own life and my own goals speculating about whom Brad was seeing or what Marcy was doing or how my aunt felt about something I did five years ago. I literally just stopped. I was done wasting my time. Trying to change people sure did make me realize how silly it is to try to change anyone or anything but *myself,* and I found way more productive things to do immediately, like meditate, write, go for a run, or work on my Personal Power.

Start to Determine What You're Worth

On average, Americans have about three to five careers in a lifetime. This is because we're constantly changing our minds and ideas about where our skills lie, what fulfills us, and how we can help others. Figuring out that I could set my own hourly rate, my own hours, and my own job title, living space, and the ability to have a bank account that wasn't in the negative numbers were all incredible revelations that I had never had before, and it made me feel awesome to have such mature goals.

It's empowering to constantly reevaluate what we're good at, and enlightening to consistently seek change. Hopefully, this makes us feel like we're worth more today than we were worth a month or even a moment ago. You're not the same person you were a decade, or even a day, ago—you don't have the same body, all of your cells are literally completely different than they were just seven years ago. This can be a daunting, confusing thought, or a totally beautiful concept to embrace.

Just Ask

Everyone is always asking for the newest business advice. How do we make more money? How do we truly take our dreams and turn them into realities? How do we get people to pay us for our talents?

How did I come to my new rate for a new job I wanted when the most I had ever made an hour in my life was ten times less?

Here's the big secret: I asked someone, and they said, "Sure."

Once again, the Bible put it best: "Ask and you shall receive." It doesn't say, "Doubt and you shall receive" or "Whine and you shall receive" or "Beg and you shall receive." It says *ask*. Just *ask*.

And trust me, even to this day, there are many people who wouldn't pay me my rate to work with me, even though my rate is much higher than when I started. That's *okay*. I don't work with those people. I work with people who know what I'm worth, or better, see my *true worth* and *encourage me to become better.*

If you want to make money with a skill you've been practicing, but you're not sure what to charge, throw a number out there. If a few people say no, think of it this way: you don't want to work with them *right now*. If you feel you are worth the amount you proposed, keep trying. Someone may take your bait. But be sure that you can deliver! The worst thing that you can do in business is waste other people's time.

There is another possibility: you may just not be good enough at your craft yet. If that's the case, make it a goal to work up to your proposed dollar amount in a month. Four weeks will give you enough time to improve upon your skills while charging an amount that people will pay. Save this money, made with your new skill, in a separate bank account. As you watch this account grow, your pride and confidence will grow along with it!

"A noble person attracts noble people, and knows how to hold on to them."

—Johann Wolfgang von Goethe (1749–1832),
Epic German Poet and Statesman, Natural Philosopher

Own Your Choices

The most important thing I ever did for myself during this time was to own my life choices. If someone asked me something, regardless of how embarrassing the answer was, or how much I felt it did not reflect my current personality, I told the truth about it. Not only did this help build my moral character from the ground up, it completely diffused any doubts that I had about "keeping the right people in my life." I knew that the people around me knew who I truly was, and were choosing to stick around. I developed an unshakable confidence about my desires.

I practiced this confidence every day, in my speech, in my business, in my relationships, and even though I was kind of winging it half the time, I finally understood the adage, "Fake it till you make it!" Oftentimes, if situations called for me to be someone, I became that person, plain and simple. This was less of a "put-on-a-mask" kind of situation, as it had been before, and more of a "finding-out-who-I-am" situation, which was what I had been seeking all along.

If you want your life to look different, if you want to see the world, or start running, or lose weight, or start a business, or write a book, or quit your job, there is only one way to get there: Do It. Putting the blame on others for your faults, or giving yourself excuses not to live the life you want, is depriving yourself of what you know you truly deserve. So whatever, whoever you want to be, put it out into the world. If you do this, people around you will follow suit. Like attracts like. People want to be around people who are like them—or better yet, people who make them better! Try it sincerely, and you'll see!

Reality:
For Those Who Can't Cope with Drugs

Reality without drugs, or any kind of distraction, is all about facing our true selves and not being afraid of what we see. This is not easy, which is why many of us spend our entire lives running from it. Not only do we all have a lot of shame and guilt deep down inside, it is also daunting to have to figure out how to change these lifelong patterns with virtually no guidebook. We're not encouraged to seek change. We're not encouraged to find ourselves, or embrace our quirks. In fact, most of my caretakers had gone through life with me just praying, wishing, and doing everything in their power to make sure I'd be "normal."

Stay Weird

I have a favorite mantra that's dear to my heart. It's one that I now live by. "Stay Weird." It's my favorite, because being weird was completely discouraged for me my whole life. *Stay Weird* totally speaks to me.

The tragedy of many people's lives is that they're incredibly afraid, and even feel terrible about things *before they happen.* Most of us have a hard time valuing what we do, especially if what we do is a natural talent, or considered creative, artistic, or out of the box. Don't you wish a manual came with these kinds of ambitions? A sort of *Bedtime Stories for Future Entrepreneurs* or *How Sheila Made a Really Good Living as a Painter* by Judy Blume?

However, that's why age-old tools like yoga, meditation, and changing state—all acts that invite us to meet ourselves—are so handy.

Ask Empowering Questions

Have you ever witnessed someone who was upset while on vacation? Haven't you seen brides have a tantrum or two on their wedding day—"the best day of their lives"? Have you allowed the bad moods of others to influence you negatively and bring you down to a basic state, even when you were in a good mood? A *basic state* is when you feel disempowered in a situation that should make you feel empowered.

The truth is, this happens to all of us. No matter where we are or how hard we are working on ourselves, what we call "problems" are day-to-day parts of life. No matter how successful or secure we become, in some way, shape, or form, they'll always be there.

Asking new, problem-solving, empowering questions is the only way to truly change our state of mind when problems arise. We need to focus on how we can make problems a positive force in our lives. When you're feeling stuck, focus on the things that empower you and reflect on the reasons why you've chosen your respective path. Try to lovingly understand why you've made the choices that you've made so that you can make better, more informed choices in the future.

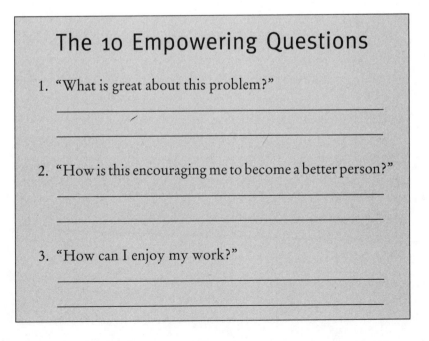

The 10 Empowering Questions

1. "What is great about this problem?"

   _____

   _____

2. "How is this encouraging me to become a better person?"

   _____

   _____

3. "How can I enjoy my work?"

   _____

   _____

4. "Who loves me? Whom do I love?"

_____

_____

5. "How can I make my work rewarding and satisfying to me and others?"

_____

_____

6. "Who supports me? Why do they support me? What am I doing right?"

_____

_____

7. "Can this event be used to create more growth in my life?"

_____

_____

8. "Where can I create perfection?"

_____

_____

9. "What am I willing to do to create the life I want?"

_____

_____

10. "How can this problem be meaningful?"

_____

_____

You Make a Difference

Without art, small businesses, big ideas, or people like you, we wouldn't have language, architecture, books, cars, computers, science, math, or any other beautiful thing—and we'd be really freaking bored.

It doesn't matter who you are or what you do, you are here for a powerful purpose, and your form of expression is valuable. Doctors aren't better than models, painters aren't better than teachers, scientists aren't better than actors. We all contribute something of worth, and anything that provides pure pleasure, like the arts, technology, or new science or inventions, is of value to society and other people. These are all ways that we can express ourselves through art. This artistic side of us is very important. Art connects us to our humanity, our soul, and one another. It provides different perspectives, teaches subtleties, and gives us multiple opportunities to learn.

You Create Your Own Future

Facing reality "sober-minded" (that is, looking at ourselves honestly) is not just about facing ourselves. Facing reality is about *becoming* ourselves.

Many people know exactly what they want to do in life, but they never do it! Why is that?

I had known what I wanted to do for years, writing, "I'll be on Broadway" in my eighth grade graduation book about "Where I'll Be in a Decade." Yet a decade later, I was a full year behind in doing it. I knew the future included a lot of makeup and a few lights, but I never really stopped to think about what that really meant for me. Where was that *Future Entrepreneurs Bedtime Stories* book when I needed it?

I knew I needed to go back there, to be that kid again. I ask you to do the same whenever you are the tiniest bit confused or discouraged about what to do next or how to create momentum in your life. Personally, I had to give up my opinionated grown-up view of "I know absolutely everything" and go back to creating possibilities. I needed to make something out of nothing. I needed to let my imagination take over, and allow it to be the only limitation that I had for the life I wanted.

Ask Your Imagination Questions

To change the way you think about yourself and your body, you need to give in to your imagination. You need to give in to unicorns and rainbows and wishes and kisses and silliness (or whatever your heart desires, but I can tell you that no matter who you are, there's a lot of silliness and even kisses in store for you once you do!). You need to imagine your small business starting, growing, and becoming something. You need to imagine yourself better, fitter, younger, and more successful and rich. You need to conjure up daily ideas of who you are at your core, and create an outer life that reflects that. You need to become the idea you had of yourself when you were a little kid.

You don't have to decide to become a fireman again, but you need to *remember why you wanted to be one*. Was it your sense of adventure? Was it the desire to help others? Was it because you admired someone who fought fires? Whatever triggered your childhood desires, use those thoughts and feelings to propel yourself into figuring out a livelihood you could truly love.

10 Questions to Trigger Your Imagination

1. What gives me a sense of wonder?

_____

_____

2. Where do I want to be in two years? Five years? Ten years?

_____

_____

3. What would get me excited to wake up in the morning?

_____

_____

4. If I were a bird, where would I fly?

_____

_____

5. If I won the lottery, what would I do with the money?

_____

_____

6. What color is my dream house?

_____

_____

7. If I could only have three possessions, what would they be?

_____

_____

8. If I had all the time in the world, what would I do?

_____

_____

9. What would I do with my life if money were no option?

_____

_____

10. If I could vacation in three spots in the next year, where would they be?

_____

_____

Don't Hate—Appreciate

The first play I ever did was *The Sound of Music*. I was seven at the time, and I reference this a lot, because I barely got cast. I was Group C, Cast C. (There was no letter after C. This made me the worst of the worst.) While the original von Trapp family in *The Sound of Music* had seven kids, Group C had about twenty kids in the show. I'm surprised anyone even came to the performance.

Despite this, I was determined to do better the next year. That summer I started voice lessons—thanks to my equally determined grandparents—and sure enough, got a solo in the next show, when I was eight. After this incident, I realized at a young age that if you work hard, you can reap the rewards in a really short amount of time.

The Sound of Music always had a special place in my heart, so at the age of twenty-four, I channeled my inner Maria and wrote a list of my favorite things.

This list included white roses, road trips, Raelie, herbs, sunsets, and Grey's smile. These were simple things, but they helped me a lot because I was doing something tremendously important to self-growth: *I was cultivating gratitude.*

I realized almost immediately—and with a sense of absolute wonder—that hate had gotten me absolutely nowhere in life, *ever*. Not one single time did getting ridiculously angry at someone else ever do me any good. It didn't build any character, it didn't help my soul, it didn't guide me on my path, it didn't help me make any friends or money; it just felt icky. I always ended up apologizing, crying, and feeling a deep sense of "I've really screwed this relationship up forever." I was tired of being triggered by everything around me, and I knew I needed to start appreciating what I had if I ever wanted to reach a point where not even grief could anger or stop me any longer.

It's important to learn to appreciate our lives in order to live them truly. Ask yourself questions about what you appreciate. Make it a ritual when you are stressed. It's especially important to hold dear the little things that you're thankful for when you feel like you can't find worth in anything, or that things are pointless. There's a reason why Rodgers and Hammerstein wrote a whole cheesy song about it. It really *works*!

10 Questions for Appreciation

1. What did I stop to admire yesterday?

   _____

   _____

2. What is great in my life right now?

   _____

   _____

3. Are there lessons I have learned from my mistakes?

   _____

   _____

4. What has my past taught me?

   _____

   _____

5. What obstacles have I overcome in my life?

   _____

   _____

6. Which things am I proud of today?

   _____

   _____

7. Who has inspired beauty for me?

   _____

   _____

8. When did I last focus on my breath?

_____

_____

9. How does my body function without me consciously working it?

_____

_____

10. For what greater purpose am I here?

_____

_____

The answers to these questions are only what we perceive to be our reality at that moment, so continue to ask yourself these questions throughout the day, and reference them whenever you are overwhelmed or stressed. They are especially helpful for restoring a sense of peace and well-being.

CHAPTER SEVEN

THE TIME YOU HAVE

"How old would you be if you didn't know how old you were?"
—Satchel Paige (1906–1982), American Baseball Player
Who Rocked the Game until the Age of Forty-Seven

My first realization that I had been breathing anxiously for years—which was surely contributing to my panic attacks, unhealthy habits, and bad moods—was not what got me to meditate every day. Not even the confirmation that everything good that I had imagined during my meditations was actually happening forced me to make this a daily practice.

Too many of us are consumed by endless, needless worry. This drains us of our natural vitality and confuses our path to wellness. I knew I had wasted a lot of time. Honestly, I didn't want *to have any time* to keep wasting time. I was twenty-five but I felt like I was seventy-five. Doctors had told me I could be paralyzed by the time I was in my thirties from arthritis. This meant, if I was lucky and could get well, I had already lived a quarter of my life. Most of it had been hazy, and then just a few years after deep memories started forming, it was spent *very* medicated.

At first, this thought deeply angered me, but then I used it to fuel my change. I wanted to banish worry and doubt about myself forever. I didn't want to be stressed out or overworked—even if I had to work hard! I thought of different ways to accomplish this. Since I was barely twenty-five and already looked like shit, my first thought was plastic surgery—or maybe Botox or the like—to fix some early signs of aging I was facing. I had friends who had relied on plastic surgery to stay young or look fit.

Warning Signs

One of the toxic friends I had once spent time with had been convinced that her breasts were "deformed" because one was bigger than the other. She saved up every penny and borrowed thousands from her family, and had an expensive breast augmentation as well as a few other surgeries when she was in her early twenties, losing almost one hundred pounds total.

It was a total transformation, and she told others that she lost this weight naturally with a raw diet. But soon after we met, she confided to me that on top of getting the surgeries, she had really been bingeing and purging her food, an eating disorder known as bulimia. The people she had lied to caught on, and they did not like it one bit.

By the time we became friends a few years later, she had major health complications as a result of her past surgeries, and told me that she was afraid to go back to the doctor because he might judge her for being bigger than she was when she went to see him the last time. The judgment that she feared from others was the reason she had gotten surgery to begin with!

Also, when she showed me the before-and-after pictures of her "deformed" breasts, I had to acknowledge that they looked, really, very normal. One was clearly a little larger than the other one, but so were mine. As far as I knew, not being completely symmetrical there was completely normal. When I told her this, she looked at me like I was crazy. "Look!" She pointed, clearly seeing something different than what I saw. "They're deformed!"

This insecurity was also reflected in our friendship. She was downright clingy and constantly doing things for attention. I confided to her that I was worried about her, but this still did not stop her. Our friendship only lasted a few short weeks, but after I stepped away, she continued to blame me and everyone around her for her misery.

She was stuck in a pattern of self-destructive behavior, and had never taught herself otherwise. This had gone on for years and taken many different forms. I had given in to this kind of behavior in the past, mostly out of guilt. But now, this kind of life served as a huge warning sign to me: *change nothing, and nothing will change.*

This had taught me that plastic surgery sometimes fixed things on the outside, but it made no effort to deal with the true cause: how we see ourselves. Not that plastic surgery was really an option for me—but it was something I wondered about for "when I got older." Honestly, I knew at the very least that my stress, my dark circles, and many of my skin problems had been caused by monotony: doing the same tasks and thinking the same negative, disempowering thoughts, every single day.

As Happy as You Want to Be

Abraham Lincoln is thought to have said, "Most folks are about as happy as they want to be." What motivated me to meditate on my health, ramp up my positive thoughts, and get in the mood to change not just some of my life, but all of my life, was one statistic, and one little sentence. First, the statistic:

We have approximately twelve thousand to sixty thousand thoughts per day.
Approximately 80 percent of our thoughts are negative or repetitive.

Next, the sentence, from the Indian mystic, guru, and spiritual teacher Osho:

"My meditation is simple. It does not require any complex practices. It is simple. It is singing. It is dancing. It is sitting silently."

Now, whether it was because the word simple appears *twice*, or whether it was because this was the first time I had ever read that "singing" was a form of "meditation," or whether this just gave me the first idea that meditation could be done everywhere, I clung to it. Likewise, I practiced it everywhere I went. Sitting, yoga, singing, dancing, taking a walk, road-tripping, and speaking with others were all opportunities for me to connect with myself. This changed everything.

It meant that I could always choose to be better. Not just for the fifteen minutes I had to meditate at the end of the day, not just when I opened myself up to conversations about health with others, not just when it was convenient. *I could be getting better all the time.*

The most remarkable thing about this timeless quote was that, when I told people that those were meditation practices, everybody understood. I mean, don't we all kind of wish we could spend our lives singing, dancing, and sitting quietly? That sounds pretty great, doesn't it? I felt that after an intense life of overstimulation, just "sitting silently," as Osho so eloquently put it, was the best meditation there was.

Your Choices

I was starting to understand that life was all about harnessing my choices, to decide what excited me and what didn't. In July 2011, before I moved, I took a road trip with Henry to Ohio, his small rural hometown, for the wedding of two of his childhood friends. I'd never road-tripped before, never been to Ohio, never left my dog, and wasn't too keen on meeting strangers (or weddings for that matter), but this journey was really fun and eye-opening. It left me feeling five years younger! This one road trip completely put my move to California into perspective and confirmed that all the steps I'd taken were in the right direction. It made everything I was doing suddenly seem like a very good decision.

The road trip to Ohio was magical. I finally experienced country life, simple living, and a real sense of adventure. From shooting my first gun to eating my first bar peanuts, I was completely enthralled. Out in the backwoods of the country, in the silence, I whispered to Henry, "What the hell is that loud noise?"

It was then we realized that I had never heard frogs before. He couldn't stop laughing about that one. City girl, indeed!

It made me even more excited about the impending cross-country road trip, and I thought about it a lot as we drove back there a few months later, our first stop on the way to California.

Still, Dad's "six months to live" stage IV cancer diagnosis was hitting me hard, and I knew I had to start harnessing my choices if I wanted to be able to deal with it, or reach my ultimate goal, which was to actually help him through it. I also wanted to take control of my own health, because cancer was an all-too-familiar word in my family, and I never wanted to have to sit there while a doctor explained my odds to me.

Changes

The idea that my breath could change or even control my thoughts and health had actually never occurred to me before, even as a scientist. I was still unconvinced that it worked that way—there must be some other explanation.

So, I did what any Westerner who begins meditating does: I stopped.

Luckily for me, I didn't stop for long.

The very next morning, I woke up unable to breathe. I was *throwing up*! It had started before my eyes even opened. I spent the rest of the day in bed with a garbage can next to my head. I had regressed about six months in my recovery from one day of not taking time to focus on solutions to my problems or relax my mind! I had gone back to thinking I could treat myself terribly, waste my time with negative thinking, and not see consequences. *Wrong!*

Well, fine, I thought. *Meditation it is!* And I drew a hot bath. I committed to myself that very night, eyes closed, entire body immersed in a scorching promise, that a meditation in the bath would become a daily practice regardless of whether or not I felt like it was helping me. This was actually an easy decision based on the toxic crap and thoughts I had put into my body before without ever thinking twice about it.

I was newly inspired to begin loving myself. It felt really good to care about myself again. The idea that I was doing something—anything—to nurture myself *was reason enough*! I knew that, even if it wasn't helping me *that very day, it couldn't possibly be hurting me.*

Pinch Yourself

Thoughts are living things. The qualities of your thoughts are what determine everything from your paycheck to your partner to your quality of life. And yet, most of us don't give our thought patterns any significance at all! I had grown up thinking that negative thoughts were a normal part of everyday life. It turned out that negative thinking was the worst disease of all. Negative thinking had drained everyone I knew, wasted a ton of time, aged everybody terribly, and had contributed to every single fight, health problem, or weak-minded action I could name.

I started to think about my negative thoughts as little pinpricks I was giving myself, or another form of self-harm. Since negative thoughts had actually been the trigger for harming myself in the past, this wasn't a far leap. I took this one step further: every time I caught myself getting immersed in negative thoughts and feelings, or wanting to act out, I would actually pinch myself.

This may sound totally absurd. Tell me about it. It was especially weird for someone who, just a few weeks prior, was pretty sure that the solution to all her problems was going to be found in an ashram, or in a single line of a single book, or in a living guru, and be something super deep and enlightening. So imagine my surprise when I found my enlightenment in *pinching myself.* It started to serve as a metaphor: *I was waking myself up from the dream of the ego.*

The Ego's Dream

Ego, in Latin, means *I*. This may explain just about everything about the ego. It is all *about us, right now*. There are no mistakes in life: only lessons. But the ego doesn't see this. All the ego sees is injustice, anger, greed, and resentment. The ego's dream is to control everything around it, all the time. And it'll steal our time any chance it gets. It always wants to be the best, brightest, most sought-after, most perfect person in the room. The ego wants us to be better than the person next to us. The ego wants to separate us, and it will convince us that this separation is real every moment that it can. The ego resists stealing directly from the person we envy, but it doesn't stop us from wasting our time going after what they have.

As much as the ego tells us that we deserve it all, it also tells us things like "We can't," "We aren't," and "We shouldn't." It's an identity of our own construction, and it's unreal. The ego hides behind the definitions of *I* simply *because it can*. It lives in a world where these kinds of thoughts about ourselves have been perfectly constructed for us.

The Unreal World

The catch? This world isn't real. Once we believe that what we have defines who we are, *we're automatically stuck*. We then live in a world where our perceptions of ourselves are totally inaccurate, because they rely on *something* or *someone else* to complete them.

We're all a part of something larger than ourselves, but we live in a world where "separateness" is the new normal. When's the last time you turned on the TV and heard someone—better yet, more than one person—talking about being made from the same material as the ground, a tree, or a rock? Or the fact that humans only have ten thousand more genes than the simple fruit fly (which has fourteen thousand genes)? Not recently, huh? But there are a lot of TV shows about who has what, who owns what, who's worth what, and who deserves what. *Why is this?*

Choices

First of all, most of us are actually choosing this kind of separateness. It's comfortable. I had spent a lot of my time in front of the

TV, wrapped up in the problems of people I would never meet, instead of fixing my own problems. I had spent my time learning what was acceptable in my society instead of learning what was acceptable in my own mind.

As much as we hate to be alone, we love being defined. It gives us a place to belong. That adage, "Why fit in when you can stand out?" resonates with most of us . . . *kind of.* Of course a part of us desperately *wants* to fit in, and is disappointed when other people reject our ideas, beliefs, passions, or even something like our fashion sense. This starts early in life, and we carry it with us, sometimes forever. We feel love in little ways: in sex, when we excel at work, when someone loves us, but we never fully experience it *from ourselves.*

This all brought me to confront the idea of why I hadn't meditated about my health before. It was the same reason I had given myself to not meditate at all in the first place. The reason was because I had never fully committed to it, I thought I was better than it, I didn't think it was "really for me," I thought it was a temporary thing I could do, and furthermore, no one had ever told me I could. But these were excuses, and I was over them.

Meditation for Your Health

The first step is to be willing to see things differently. If you're willing to do this, everything—*I mean everything*—will change for you. Once you change, it is not a matter of *if* your life changes, it's all about *how* your life changes.

Breathing unconsciously for years had actually sincerely messed me up. It had given me a shallow, panicked living mechanism that I carried everywhere, into everything. This had—for sure—translated into shallow, panicked coping mechanisms. I could barely make myself breathe correctly in real life, even after a month of daily meditation. I consistently caught myself breathing incorrectly, and was constantly scolding myself, but lovingly. I had been to decades of vocal lessons, lying on my back and singing scales—sometimes entire songs—with my hand on my diaphragm. In, out. In, out. I had learned this lesson at a very early age, and *this was the outcome*?

Applying It

Sure, I had learned proper, conscious breathing by the time I was eight years old, but what had I done with it? Not much, unless it was right before an audition. We can have all the knowledge in the world, but if we don't apply it, we're no better off.

The truth was, despite learning the lesson, I had only committed it to one thing: singing. My voice. I never applied breathing properly to everyday life, even though I knew all about it.

Applying my lessons properly, and throughout my life, was my first step to committing to my "timeless" meditation practice.

Commitment

I realized suddenly that *it is our commitment to looking and feeling well that counts*—and putting our thoughts in a healthy place is the first step to this commitment. We can *want* health all day long, but it is not until we are *committed to health* and *act on it* that our thoughts manifest into anything we can recognize. No matter where we are in life, this is an important step to staying well, young, and vibrant. I was super psyched that I had figured this out! It meant that, if this worked, *I had all the tools I needed—right in my own mind—to combat age, disease, time, and years of unhealthy habits.*

Someone Else's Agenda

This is where I met my first roadblock, as we often do once a change takes place in us. The second I committed to this method of healing, someone else's agenda showed up.

Remember the unhappy former friend I had, who was all about complaining and getting plastic surgery to fix her problems? Even though I had not spoken with her in years, she immediately popped up once I made this solid commitment to myself. And boy, was her resentment level as high as ever! Once she learned that I was getting well, she discouraged it in every way she could think of. Things like telling me to go back on medication, gossiping to my friends, discouraging my healthiest behaviors (like going to the gym or on a hike) were all part of her program. No matter what direction I headed in toward wellness, she couldn't stand it.

It wasn't that my unhappy former friend even believed I was truly doing the wrong thing. It was clear to me that her judgments were coming from an insecure, hurt place. If she wanted to feel hurt, there was nothing I could do. Apologies hadn't worked. She saw me getting better, happier, and well and it drove her crazy. This happens. I see this happen to my clients, my family, and my friends all the time. Some people just can't stand to watch you succeed.

Has this ever happened to you? You make one big, solid commitment to yourself and someone—sometimes someone you least expect—constantly questions or tries to undermine what you're doing? This behavior is a form of resentment. I sensed *mass insecurity*, because I had lived in that haze myself for a very long time. I was learning that the people following someone else's agenda were not the people I wanted in my life. Following someone else's agenda and opinion is *comfortable*, and I was trying to surround myself with *leaders*. Leaders are people who make themselves uncomfortable constantly in order to improve. I did not need more followers as friends.

Remember, you are *your own* person. Being your own person means pushing yourself beyond your comfort zone. It means that the choices you make are yours and yours alone. Other people will see those choices and ultimately have their judgments about them, but unless those judgments are encouraging you on your path, they really don't have a place on your journey.

Don't let someone else impose themselves upon your life. If they discourage you from growth, if they prevent you from following your dreams, they have no place in your life. Sure, as human beings, we all seek approval, but if this "approval" is coming in the form of conforming to someone else's whims, or changing to fit a hater's standard of who you should be, it's not the type of approval that you want. It won't propel you forward.

When this unhappy person started imposing herself on my life, I realized that I wasn't interested in having friends who loved petty gossip, or turning their backs on others. If people were willing to entertain anything she may have said about me or think any less of me because of it, they also were not the people I wanted in my life. *This might make my circle of friends smaller but at least it'll stop me from wasting my time.* Furthermore, it occurred to me that all of these people were wasting *their time.* They didn't *know me*, and now they *never would.*

The Most Important Thought

I turned back to my breath. This was the most important thought that had occurred to me socially thus far. It allowed me to completely drop the idea that I needed anyone's approval to live my life. It was hard not to care that other people bought in to so much bullshit, but I knew I had to let it go.

So, I focused on my own health, my own breathing, and my own improvements. I focused on my breathing and posture *constantly, even if it looked or felt silly to do.* I knew that if what other people were doing to stay young, fit, and happy wasn't working, that I might have to just invent my own way. I was okay with that, and already had a great basis that had worked for all my other life changes: *changing my thoughts.* I was determined to change my philosophy on aging, on stress, and on health immediately along with my commitment to stay off pharmaceutical drugs.

Antiaging

It was that night that I started my "antiaging" meditations. I called them this then because—let's face it—*that's what I was trying to get out of doing them.* I call them that now because *that is what they've truly accomplished for me.*

That same night, I compiled a list of proper excuses I had given myself about why I had not meditated on looking better and feeling younger before, so that if I ever met one of these excuses again, I would recognize it. My aches and pains were at the top of the list of things I wanted to solve, yet I had invested almost no time into alternative treatment for them besides herbs. Although taking herbs and salt baths did help me incredibly, I really didn't concentrate on the healing process with meditations as much as I should have. My daily meditations had hardly focused on physical aging or health for more than a few minutes. I'd always been concentrated on relieving the pain or the source of discomfort, but now I wanted to shift my focus, to feel completely dis-ease free, youthful, and lovely.

So, whenever I got frustrated during my healing process, I would concentrate on feeling well and vibrant, and relax. Instead of focusing on my digestion, or my joint pain, I started to see light throughout *my whole body.* Then, I carried this feeling of lightness into everything I did.

I began to come up with personal exercises for slowing down my own process of aging, which I was desperate to reverse. A life of excess had definitely left its mark.

I encourage you wholeheartedly to meditate and relax when you find yourself up against a roadblock in your process, or feel confused about where to go next in your journey. Meditation is meant to inspire you, as well as provide a clear-cut trail to your own personal path to wellness.

I meditate in conjunction with taking herbs, such as ashwagandha, sage, and fenugreek, that have antiaging properties, like flavonoids and antioxidants to combat free radicals.

Meditation for a Healthy Existence

Sit up straight in your chair with your feet firmly on the ground.

Breathe in deeply through your nose and out through your mouth.

Breathe In: I am absolute existence.

Breathe Out: I am free from dis-ease.

Breathe In: I am absolute existence.

Breathe Out: I am free from dis-ease.

Breathe In: Thank you for reminding me of what is real.

Breathe Out: Thank you for reminding me of what is real.

Open your eyes and write down whatever free-flowing feelings you experience after this meditation.

Movement

I have absolutely no appreciation for the word *exercise*. Exercise sounds like work. It sounds like I need to suit up and plop in a DVD. It sounds like I'm going to have to buy something. More so, it sounds like it's gonna take me all day.

I prefer the word *movement*. Movement means something different to me every day, but it is my number one natural cure for everything from stiff muscles to depression. And I don't dread doing it.

Often when we feel down, our tendency is to loaf around and hope it passes. This method stagnates our blood, tenses our muscles, and numbs our aesthetic-loving and ever-coping minds. Think about how much exercise you're getting while just walking that you're not even really thinking about! Your arms sway, your breathing steadies, your back muscles relax, and your legs are moving while you walk! Without natural pleasures, it's hard to get back to a place of being present and aware.

All forms of media—news, entertainment, movies, television—are, in a way, dead things. They've already been created, edited, stripped, voiced over, mass-produced, and watched by millions of others. Your walks, your hikes, your bike rides—those are all YOU, and no one will see them the way you do! Studies show that even ten minutes of walking in the sunlight per day can dramatically improve your mood, balance your circadian rhythms, and help you get better rest.[15]

"You never know what you can do until you have to do it."
—Betty Ford (1918–2011), First Lady of the USA,
Breast Cancer Survivor, Women's Rights Activist

Your Vocabulary

Does the word *vocabulary* remind you of those dreaded tests in grade school, sitting at your desk, sounding out words as your teacher read them aloud to the class? They were definitely no fun (unless you were dorky like me; I kind of loved them . . .), but those long hours spent memorizing words and sounding out syllables were not all in vain! Vocabulary, when used with empowering thought-tactics, can be incredibly powerful in creating your own personal reality. Thought-tactics are devices we use in everyday life to switch our reality, using our vocabulary. And they make me really grateful that I had stayed alert and interested during vocab class, no matter how dorky I looked.

A thought-tactic might include switching out the word "hate" from our vocabulary for something different. Instead of saying, "I hate those pants!" we might say, "I don't favor those pants" or "These pants don't strike my fancy."

These may seem like absurd or unnatural ways of speaking, but humor yourself and just try them out. Even laugh at yourself if you have to! Your vocabulary is the one thing that's been up to you *all along*. Have you chosen a rich one or a poor one?

Transformation

Our vocabulary has the power to create what is important to us in a moment. Instantaneously, our ideas about who we are can be transformed, simply by transferring from poor thinking to *thoughtful abundance.*

Thoughtful abundance occurs when we finally have our internal vocabularies straightened out. We don't sound wiser or better or smarter than anyone else—we just make more sense.

This was the first time people went from seeing me as a pretentious private school kid to seeing me as a relatable adult who might actually kind of have some of her shit figured out. *Seriously*. People perked up at what I said and we both went home and thought about it. They took my advice. They bounced ideas off me. I was making more sense. I was thinking more clearly, and getting much greater insight into other people's lives. The next time I spoke to someone was always filled with excitement. Our conversations would always start with "I thought about something you said, and I've been thinking . . ."

These exciting conversations had almost made me hesitant to leave New York, on the one hand. I was finally connecting to people I had always butted heads with before, including people in my family, and I was making new and important friends. I knew, though, that if these people were meant to be in my life, they would be.

I was also learning some very important lessons. The most major one was that I didn't have to know everything about everything to connect with someone, as long as I kept an open mind. I could give good advice about someone's marriage, even though I'd never been married. I could guide someone through a doctorate program, even though I wasn't a PhD. I could help a business make good financial decisions, even though I wasn't yet a business owner. I was gaining insight, and it was a really powerful way to share my thoughtful abundance.

Meditations for Thoughtful Abundance

Sit up straight in your chair with your feet firmly on the ground.

Breathe in deeply through your nose and out through your mouth.

Breathe In: I am ever-mindful.

Breathe Out: I accept thoughtful abundance.

Breathe In: I am ever-mindful.

Breathe Out: I accept thoughtful abundance.

Breathe In: Thank you for this breath.

Breathe Out: Thank you for reminding me of what is real.

Carrying the Tools

The idea that I carried all of the tools I needed inside of me all along—if I just read the right books, thought the right things, said the right words, and practiced the right actions—was incredibly inspiring, reassuring, and rewarding.

I was tired of trying to fit in. I wanted to stand out in a way that other people responded to. I didn't want people to "want to be" me or even "look up to" me. Instead I wanted people to see and feel a certain *something* around me, an aura that in turn inspired them to be the best version of themselves that they could be. I wanted to be able to do this everywhere, with anyone, and use it to accomplish anything I really put my mind to.

Yogananda says, "The affirmation seed must be a living one, free from the defects of doubt, restlessness, or inattention. It should be sewn in the mind and the heart with concentration, devotion, and peace. . . . It should be watered with deep, fresh repetition and boundless faith."

I found this "fresh repetition and boundless faith" in my everyday activities and every time I confirmed this for myself, it became easier to do so. Much like my old negative thoughts had a constant place on the shelf, these new, empowering, positive thoughts were finding their place in my life, front and center. They were "free from defects of doubt, restlessness, and inattention" and they definitely had root in my heart.

Whether I was on the subway, getting shortchanged at the grocery store, booking a job, seeing a friend, or missing a bus, I felt an overwhelming sense of peace and tranquility that I could only explain with the adoption of these time-grasping exercises. Also, the more peace I felt, *the less I seemed to need it*! People responded to my outward glow immediately, and were less likely to swindle, shortchange, leave, or otherwise screw me over in the first place. It was, in a word, miraculous.

It occurred to me that just six months ago, I had literally been hacking off my arm from pain and self-pity. Now, I was living my dreams, and on the cusp of even bigger things that I could only imagine. I tried another meditation practice at night to remind myself of all of the power I carried within myself to solve my problems.

Meditation for Building Your Tools

Sit up straight in your chair with your feet firmly on the ground or in a lotus position.

Breathe in deeply through your nose and out through your mouth.

Breathe In: I am empowered.

Breathe Out: I carry all my tools.

Breathe In: I am empowered.

Breathe Out: I carry all my tools.

Breathe In: Thank you for reminding me of who I am.

Breathe Out: Thank you for reminding me of what is real.

Repeat your affirmations for at least seven breaths. Avoid mechanical repetition in your mantras or your daily affirmations and meditations. The time you have is extremely precious. Repeat your affirmations firmly, with intensity and sincerity, until you feel the power from within moving you forward. One command, one strong urge from within, will be enough to change the very cells of your body, and move your soul to perform your own daily miracles in a way that will improve your health, clear your path, decrease signs of aging, and truly heal your body.

CHAPTER EIGHT

WISDOM: THE GREATEST CLEANSER

"The great pleasure in life is doing what people say you cannot do."

—Walter Bagehot (1826–1877),
British Journalist, Essayist, Businessman, Epic Beard Sporter

All of the bottoms I had hit throughout my life had been the catalyst for this incredible change and transformation, and I was grateful for them all. Looking back, I wouldn't have done a single thing differently: I saw where each action had led me. Each and every pill, terrible decision, rendezvous with near-death, and depressing thought had all pushed me to a point of no return. It was Wellness, or Bust! It's amazing how quickly you adjust once you've really made up your mind about something.

It was October 2011. Just ten months previously I had been at the funeral of one of my best friends. Nine months previously I had tried to take my own life, and ended my three-year abusive relationship. Eight and a half months ago I had come off of all the medication I had been on for over a decade. Seven months ago I had made meditation a daily practice in my life, and repeatedly reaped its rewards. Three months ago I had taken my first road trip ever, and fallen in love with the idea of traveling. Two and a half months ago I had put the down payment on an apartment over three thousand miles away from home, in a city that I had never been to before, then swallowed the idea that I might lose Dad to cancer in just half a year.

Then, just one day before my road trip, we wrapped up my first movie and I had my first—tiny, but fueling—feature film role under my belt. *What a year it had already been!* I packed up a 2007 Ford Fusion with everything I owned, said my good-byes to my family, and was on the road with Henry and $300 to my name. This was, seriously, one of the most fun and incredible decisions I had ever made!

The road trip was eye-opening, beautiful, wonderful, and magical. Vast, open space, strangers, friendships, new places, and brand-new things awaited me, and the romantic in me was totally enthralled. I wanted to settle everywhere I went, but was also eager to get to California and make my home there.

We didn't make too many sightseeing stops, but when we did, luck found us. We met wonderful, kind strangers, found quaint places, ate amazing food, made great friends, and above all else, I was incredibly inspired to start taking photographs again, a hobby I had put down for a good few months after Grey's death.

I had a camera in my hand just about every time I wasn't driving, snapping away. I really enjoyed this aspect of capturing my journey, and wrote in my journal: *In love with photography. Holding a camera is the closest I have felt to home in years. Also, time is going backward. I watched the sun set over and over again, as we crossed three different states going west today! Every single thing about these moments is life-changing!*

Maya

Again and again throughout my long drives through foreign states, I thought about the concept of *maya*. I had read about it in Yogananda's teachings, and for the first time, it finally made sense to me.

In *Scientific Healing Affirmations*, Yogananda writes, "Maya is the law of duality, or oppositional states: it is thus an unreal world that veils the truth."

Maya was a limited physical and mental illusion. It was the reality that I had lived in all along: trapped, overconscious of the wrong parts of myself. It was that which was only true *for now*: fleeting things like pleasures, irrational decisions, and even pain were all a part of it. As I felt the wind on my face somewhere in Texas, things started to fall into place in a way I had never experienced before. I was what they call "piercing the veil" of maya's delusion.

Wisdom Is the Greatest Cleanser

In some Hindu literature, maya has a dual sense. I thought of maya as a blurry film over reality, slightly warping my vision of everything, and making the world less beautiful than it truly was. However, it was also a film that I could clean off whenever I wanted to in order to see things more clearly. It is said that when the "veil is pierced" and the separate realities are recognized, the knowledge of maya can be a form of magic. Using the knowledge of maya to my advantage was my ultimate goal. It was one thing to know about all this stuff, but I wanted to *practice* it. I wanted to live in my own world of peace, *while also being able to deal with the real world around me.*

Swami Sri Yukteswar, Yogananda's guru, said, "Wisdom is the greatest cleanser." Although we are all subject to change and some limitations, tapping into our greater wisdom about ourselves is the only way to free ourselves of an anxiety-filled life. This is exactly what I was trying to do through meditations and my constant search for wisdom. I finally had control over my inner dialogue, I had figured out how to follow my dreams, and I was beginning to find my bliss.

Clouds

My first bliss-filled experience was in Albuquerque. Henry and I had driven into New Mexico super late the night before, and as we soared over a long stretch of dark highway, I remember thinking, *I can't see a thing. What does this place look like?* The air was heavy with warmth and possibility. As we pulled into a small hotel parking lot, my eyes adjusted to the darkness. There, in the distance, were the biggest clouds I had ever seen. I was so excited for the morning that I spent practically all of that night awake, restless for my day trip to Arizona and then to my new apartment in Hollywood!

I woke up very early and pulled the curtains back just a peek. I was totally astonished at what I saw in the dusty haze of dawn.

The clouds from the night before weren't clouds at all! They were mountains! Beautiful, sky-high, pink, purple, majestic mountains as far off into the dusky distance as I could see! I had never witnessed anything like them before! These big, gorgeous, magical, mystical, gentle giants were everywhere. They dotted my eyesight in every direction, and I was so anxious to explore that I woke Henry up, begging him to take a trip with me somewhere. He had a strange twinkle in his eye.

"Just wait until we get to California," he laughed at me. "This is *nothing*."

I *couldn't believe it*. I had absolutely never seen anything so beautiful before and spent the entire rest of my day looking up. Not the way I had seen people look up in New York City, staring slack-jawed, in awe at the tiny pieces of coy sky peeking out between the impossibly tall buildings. This was different: it was a connection I had never felt before to the open terrain and the great, rolling landscape. I was deeply in love with nature, with the warmth, with the desert, with the feeling of my toes in the sand. I was totally hooked.

As If

This was the first day my imagination really took off in regard to what California, and my future, had in store for me. I was finally getting excited, not just about leaving New York, or seeking adventure, but I was also finally getting excited *about where that adventure might lead me.*

That very day, I started to constantly act *as if* good things were already happening in my new life. I expected daily miracles. I went to bed *as if* I were going to wake up bright and early and tackle the day. I handled problems *as if* I already knew how to solve them. I spoke to people *as if* they were already excited and responsive. I felt happy, *as if* every day were Christmas. I acted *as if* good things were going to come my way.

And they did! *As if* went from being a catchphrase in *Clueless* to the two powerful words that were beginning to shape my life and help me find my bliss in everything. As we headed for Arizona (and Henry's family), I acted *as if* we were going to get there safe and sound, and everything was going to work out, no matter what happened.

Arizona

The drive from New Mexico to Arizona happened beautifully, without a hitch. The landscape was some of my favorite yet. Going through the bland flatlands of the middle of the country had gotten a little ridiculous for me, personally. By the time we were in Oklahoma I had become kind of bored and every new turn was more sketchy than the last. Henry and I found ourselves staying with his former college roommate, who was deep into a bad heroin addiction. To escape possibly having everything we owned robbed for dope, we found a cozy place to crash for breakfast. (Side note: After going to rehab, starting daily meditation practices, and cleaning up his diet, that friend is now sober and one of our dearest and sweetest compadres.) I could see why it was hard for him to stay sober here. By 8:00 a.m., most of the people around me were on their second beer.

"Where the fuck are we?" I asked, over some true country eggs.

"Oh, right," Henry said. "You've never been to the South."

All in all, the South totally gave me the wrong vibes. Between the cowboy hats, Southern drawl, casual gun laws, diagnosable alcoholism, and thick accents, I was beyond ready to get onto Western soil.

Arizona was a blessing. I had considered moving there when researching places to begin with, but the job market didn't appeal to me at all. The place totally tripped me out in all the best ways, though. I was constantly in awe of the vast landscapes, gorgeous sunsets, agreeable weather, and big, fluffy clouds. The sky constantly remained a perfect baby blue, the likes of which I had barely seen in photographs. The dry air also did wonders for my back, soothing my aches and pains almost immediately in a way nothing else ever had.

Also, certain places that we drove by definitely possessed an energy that you could feel, even from a few miles away. Always a "sacred land" skeptic, this idea of sacred spaces on earth actually started to really grow on me. The orange mountains, fiery sunsets, and baby blue skies were truly calming. I suddenly felt more grounded, more centered, and more attuned to everything around me; I found myself connecting with nature for the first time in my life.

We rested a few days in Arizona, but a huge part of me just couldn't wait to get back on the road. Whether it was exploring, driving around, hiking, sightseeing, or finding a good place to meditate at dawn, I made little rituals for myself every day to get outside now that I had absolutely no excuses.

I was also still acting *as if*. *As if* I weren't in any rush to get to my tiny Hollywood studio apartment. Henry and his family could all tell that my heart longed for my new home, and after a few days at Henry's folks' house in Arizona, we set out for California.

Little Pleasures

When we have to choose between growing or staying safe, most of us choose safety. Other people—a spouse, friend, parent, or sibling—can trigger the most profound feelings in us, and it's easier to blame these people for our mistakes rather than to face ourselves and take the rap for our bad decision-making or stubbornness. Often the more we try to coerce ourselves into changing, the more deeply entrenched in our habits we become. This may at least partially account for the reason most people who diet gain their weight back. Learning how to treat ourselves well is the missing link to finding this balance. When we learn to find that balance, we can rapidly build self-esteem, and we immediately begin to appreciate the little things that show up in beautiful, tangible ways.

Finding pleasure in the simple things in life was becoming extremely important to my own sense of well-being and how I was treating myself. It was constantly reaffirmed to me that my sense of happiness depended on me and only me. I learned it in all kinds of hard ways. When my source of happiness relied on someone else, for instance, I realized I was immediately totally screwed.

Since we're trying to move ahead in our personal growth, which can take some time, we don't need to rush into doing anything. Whether it's finding new work or a different place to live that we love, nothing should ever be rushed—it'll happen when you're ready, or sometimes when the Universe is ready. Just focus on the little things that bring you joy. This is another way of cultivating gratitude, a topic we've touched on a bit before.

Cultivating Little Pleasures

If you found five minutes every morning to meditate and affirm the positive things in your life to yourself for the next year, you'd have 1,825 minutes of meditation under your belt! (And I'd totally find five minutes to brag about that too, if I were you!) Just a few minutes when you wake up in the morning to say, "I am thankful for who I am" or "I am here to greet this wonderful day" really, truly add up. Finding quiet surroundings to appreciate nature and practice my affirmations was integral to my healing and self-discovery. Simply noticing what you connect with and what you are grateful for every day—and how that changes—will absolutely change you.

Nowadays, I don't even take a nap without a little affirmation or a future-focused meditation before I drift off to sleep. These good thoughts not only impact my dreams, they impact my rest! Getting good rest is essential to functioning properly, and thinking good thoughts before you let your unconscious brain take over is the only way to have control over those unconscious thoughts and ultimately, your life!

Free Your Mind

I started every morning with a long, hot bath. If I had suggested taking a bath in the morning to most people I had lived with previously, they would have looked at me sideways. I know baths were something I grew up thinking of as a pre-bedtime ritual, not something I did right as I woke up. But this idea that I was capable of healing any way I wanted was still so present in my mind that I found myself embracing new ways to get well at every turn.

Then, I found a quiet place to think. Even if this was a corner of a room no one was in or a part of the yard that was all my own, it helped me to free my mind of all doubts and worries, aches and pains, and begin the day fresh and new. Freeing your mind of doubts and worries in the morning clears the way for proper thinking throughout your whole day. It leaves tons of room for better decision-making, better coping, and creating a better you!

Finding Sounds That Heal You

Of all the things, among gun laws, bullying, and depression, that the media could have reported on when Eric Harris and Dylan Klebold murdered twelve students and one teacher in the 1999 Columbine High School massacre, they blamed music. The majority of the blame was directed at bands like KMFDM and Rammstein, or the popular goth musician Marilyn Manson. Manson defended himself, as well as attacked the news media for their irresponsible coverage. When asked by director Michael

PART TWO: STAY WEIRD

Moore what he would have said to the boys, Manson answered, "I wouldn't have said a single word to them. I would have *listened to what they have to say, and that's what no one did.*"

Music may not have the power to make two boys decide to take drastic negative action, but it definitely has enough influence to spark massive media coverage. And I had *definitely* identified with punk, hardcore, emo, grunge, screamo, gothic, and depressing music in my darker hours. I'd repeat these songs over and over. Now, I found no solace at all in these same songs or lyrics.

Did you ever hear a song in the car, in the store, or in an elevator and then find yourself singing it moments later, only to wonder where you'd heard it? Finding sounds that heal you is so important, because these sounds really do get stuck in our heads! Without consciously choosing what you listen to, or trying to improve what you're choosing to hear, it's incredibly hard to stay focused on improvement in your life. A very strong mind is the basis for overcoming any problem we face in life, even extremely difficult health problems. Music can set us up for achieving a very strong mind.

You are a product of whatever you are putting into your mind (or in your ears in this case). Music has the capability to soothe us and calm us down in just a moment. It can inspire us, heal us, or make us smile.

As an example, I started chanting. At the end of the Beatles song "Across the Universe," the lyrics that repeat *"Jai guru deva, om"* over and over were the first daily chant that I started. It means, "I give thanks to my guru/teacher (amen)."

The next chant I repeated every morning to myself was *"Om Namah Shivaya"* (ohm nah-mah shi-vye-ya). This means "I am saturated with light." This is a phrase I used to connect to my bliss and find the divinity inside myself. It was the chant I used to envision my true purpose. There are many chants and mantras that you can start doing for health, wellness, love, prosperity, wealth, or whatever you desire.

If it's easier to connect, some of these chants can of course be in your own comfortable language. One of my favorite chants is in

English, based on a chant from Yogananda, which I have slightly modified for the purpose of this book, as his language can get kind of dated.

Affirmation for Connection

Sit up straight in your chair with your feet firmly on the ground.

Breathe in deeply through your nose and out through your mouth.

Breathe In: I think my life to flow.

Breathe Out: I know my life to flow.

Breathe In: The little cells are drinking.

Breathe Out: Their tiny mouths all are thinking.

Breathe In: The little cells are drinking.

Breathe Out: Their tiny mouths all are thinking.

I love this little meditation because I can picture my cells drinking up the oxygen and life force around me and smiling as I take in light.

List Your Gratitude

I have whole journals full of funny little lists next to longer prose or poems. Nowadays, picking them up and opening them to a random page never fails to make me smile. Some pages say things like *Rainbows* and *Baby pandas* or *The fact that I got out of bed today*. Some are perfectly categorized and numbered, some are scrawled in half-script with no date. They're my *Gratitude Lists*, and they got me off my butt and into high gear!

Most people *want* to do awesome things every day, but they're faced with the Big R: Resistance. We pick this up as children: when we don't want to do something, we resist it in every way we can. Whether it's crying, screaming, fighting, or throwing a tantrum, unless this kind of behavior is dealt with directly and managed well by our parents (and it very often is *not*) we carry this unconscious behavior into our adulthoods. It's actually become a very acceptable way to act.

My journals used to be filled with self-hatred, confusion, and negative thoughts. That's exactly what had sent me to a psychiatrist at thirteen years old in the first place! Most of us only make one kind of list: to-do lists. Replacing these kinds of habits and making daily lists of what you're grateful for, instead of a list of things *you have to do*, will encourage you to focus on the positive, amazing, small pleasures in your life instead of on the crazy crap!

Tips for Your Gratitude Lists

HANDWRITE YOUR LIST

Think about how many things you type in a day. Most of them have been school-related, personal, work-related, or stress-related, right?

Handwriting your gratitude list not only gives you the tools you need to explore yourself, but doing it by hand also gives you the kinesthetic experience of fulfilling your goals. It's also a complete dissociation from typing, which we all do so much of every day, to the point where we may have many unconscious anxieties associated with doing it. Handwriting your gratitude list works on a cellular level, and is also a slower process than typing or texting. It becomes a second way to reference and reaffirm your growth.

BE REALISTIC

Taking your gratitude seriously is important. Being realistic is also important. If you write even one thing, you've done your job. You don't have to be inspired to write pages upon pages—some days are just plain hard. Start with "I am grateful for . . ." Even if it ends with "I am grateful for sitting here" or "I am grateful for writing this," it's a very important step in the right direction.

FAKE IT TILL YOU MAKE IT!

Some days you might write without feeling an ounce of gratitude. That's okay! Just do it, and try not to get discouraged. Smile, even if you're crying. Write, even if you're tired. These acts alone are ways to affirm your personal wellness, and will absolutely put your mind and body on a track to feeling better.

When your number one goal in life is to get *results*, you'll do just about anything to get wherever you're trying to go. Whether it's putting on weight (like healthy muscle mass) or losing weight (for those who struggle with diet or exercise), remember that *your body leads your results*.

Morning Dancing

The word "dancing" was always, well . . . *daunting*. I am not, by any stretch of the imagination, a dancer. Even as a mixed girl, I can barely twerk any better than Miley Cyrus. So if this little practice seems daunting, I feel you. Believe me. But it's truly changed my life, so I encourage you to keep an open mind.

I started dancing every morning. I moved in whatever way I felt like, to whatever I cared to listen to. Even if I had to put headphones in, lock the bathroom door, and go nuts in front of the mirror for a few minutes, I figured it out. This morning dancing not only loosened my body from years of wear, tear, and stress, it made me *feel* free. No one judged me. I didn't judge myself, or check myself, or do anything but have fun.

This made me a calmer, more patient, and loving person, and I noticed changes immediately. For instance, on my first day of morning dancing, I experienced some awesome results that surprised me. I had just finished losing my shit and was retying my messy bun, stretching and sipping a smoothie. I felt very inspired, so I sat down on my meditation pillow with my pen and journal.

I made a list of behaviors about myself I simply didn't like and wanted to change. One of the top things I wanted to change was, as I plainly wrote it, "Not to go straight for the jugular every time I fight with someone." I started practicing this immediately, being more kind and understanding in my approach, talking out my feelings, truly listening to others.

I noticed results instantly. When I acted different, the people I used to fight with *thought of me* a little differently. Then, the fights stopped altogether. There was *nothing left in me that would fight back with anyone*. I had nothing to prove.

Sooner than I ever expected, I started to attract the kind of people I didn't have to argue with *at all*. This then attracted an immense amount of love into my life. When you are kind to someone else, you give them the space to be kind to you. When you radiate love, you attract people who have their antennae up to receive love. And I was being more loving. So Love was attracting Love.

When I read this list over months later, I had to laugh. It had never even occurred to me that I wouldn't be fighting with anyone in my life: *I had simply wanted to stop being as mean as I could to people I loved right off the bat.*

When I slowed down, I stopped doing clumsy things, I stopped making dumb mistakes, and, most important to me, I stopped hurting people's feelings.

"See your mind for what it is—nature's greatest gift."
—Robin S. Sharma (1965–Present),
Author of *The Monk Who Sold His Ferrari*

Practice Morning Dancing

Step 1: The night before, I would choose a playlist of four or five songs that made me feel really good. It doesn't matter if they're super cheesy, incredibly pop-y ultra trendy, or simply guilty-pleasure songs; put them on there.

> **Step 2:** In the morning, I drank four glasses of water and had a smoothie. While waiting for breakfast to cook, I put the playlist on.
> **Step 3:** I lost my shit. Seriously. I'd just do whatever dance moves came to mind. Sometimes in my underwear, or a robe, or with a face mask on. Whatever it was I had to do, I got all my energy out. I jumped up and down. I sang along loudly. I'd grab a hairbrush and pretend I was singing in front of a million people. What-*ever* got me up, encouraged me, and forced me to be physically active, I did it!

Being Your Bliss

Logan Pearsall Smith said,

"There are two things to aim at in life:
First, to get what you want.
After that, to enjoy it."

I was getting what I wanted at every turn, for the first time *ever*! I was very happy with my decisions, even if some of them were totally out of my comfort zone. The idea that each and every morning looked different and exciting was changing a lot *in itself*. Bliss was not something I was searching for: it was something I was growing, weeding, and cultivating every single day, like my lavender plants. Dancing, singing, traveling, being, meditating, doing yoga, loving, and speaking *were* my happiness.

You believe in your bliss when you believe in yourself. Confidence in your abilities, gratitude, shaking things up, and creating a different perception of growth are all great ways to start recognizing that your happiness exists in both the simple, everyday things, as well as the big successes.

There is no success without emotional success. After years of spending my mornings rushing to work on an empty stomach and shoving a bunch of pills in my mouth, then trying to keep my eyes open for the rest of the day, mornings spent dancing, meditating, and focusing on my goals and gratitude were refreshing, amazing, and life-changing!

Although you can do this anytime during the day—and should do it as much as you can—this silly little exercise in the morning and before bed at night will get you in tune with yourself, your body, and your fitness level. There were some mornings when I felt so energized after doing my morning dance routine and writing my gratitude list that I immediately went for a four-hour hike afterward, and then there were some days where I was totally breathless and shaking while pouring myself more water. Our bodies change each and every day, and this is a great way to connect regardless of where we are on the fitness scale!

As you move through your day, take this idea of movement with you. Awareness, grace, and just being thankful for your ability to move in this way are all great steps to sticking to your new morning routine!

California

It was late, and the second we crossed over the border from Arizona to California, my face broke out in a huge grin. *Home*, I thought. *I'm home.*

I will never forget my first late-night drive into Los Angeles. The lights, the warmth, the smell, the highways, and the cute little suburban houses that dotted the streets all appealed to me, *a lot*. There was a warm glow to everything that I just loved. And the *palm trees*! I had never seen so many palm trees in my entire life! I loved each and every one. They reminded me of my days as a young girl playing Malibu Barbie. I had literally imagined this, had dreamed of palm trees lining my street the way that some girls dream of their weddings or their dream house—and here I was! *Maktub*, indeed!

I would have told you that in my first week, even the smog of LA had me head over heels. I was just in love. California was different than what I had been used to in New York, different than what I had seen on the road trip, and different from anywhere I had ever traveled to. Our first stop was for a bite to eat, and I remember looking around thinking, *God damn! Everyone is beautiful!*

We were at an In-N-Out. I had absolutely no idea what I was in for.

Beliefs

Just a few years earlier, I had been sitting in the driver's seat of my ex-boyfriend's car, making manic plans to move to California with him. We talked for hours—for days—about it, *but we never took any action.* I didn't do an ounce of research. We never did anything except fight. Turns out, we couldn't even figure out how to go to dinner together.

I had finally done something I wasn't sure I was ever going to be capable of doing. As I drove down the Pacific Coast Highway for the first time, I took a tremendous amount of pride in the last ten months of my life, and all of my accomplishments. A part of me realized that my entire life—from calling my grandparents at six years old that night my mother overdosed in front of me, to every Alateen meeting where I shared my feelings, to every psychologist's appointment, to venting my frustrations in writing, to going on medication, to every fight with a loved one, to every late rehearsal, to falling into and out of abusive patterns and relationships, to getting sober and moving—had all *set me up* for wellness, *better than having known all the answers all along would have!*

I realized that the many things that led up to this decision, this relationship with myself, had started out with venting, and now I was purifying. I had been extracting, and now I was cleansing. I had been experiencing outbursts, and now I was experiencing deep catharsis.

I was just starting, and I was so, so excited! With wisdom as my greatest cleanser and my bliss under my belt, I tackled the next obstacle: changing what was on the outside to match what I was doing on the inside.

Whether it's finally making the leap, and giving into that positive voice at the back of your mind, adapting the wisdom of your greatest mentor into your life, you are in complete control of your destiny and your own bliss. This sisterhood of wisdom and bliss is what will ultimately heal you and propel you on the right path. I can't tell you what your physical destiny is, but as far as I'm concerned, neither can a doctor. Medical professionals can hypothesize a possible outcome, based on genetics or your personal history, but no one can tell you what you're destined to weigh, that you're definitely going to get diabetes, that you're incapable of exercise, or whatever your perceived medical limitations are. The answer does lie in a fun place, though. That's right: back to you, love!

PART THREE: LIVE WELL

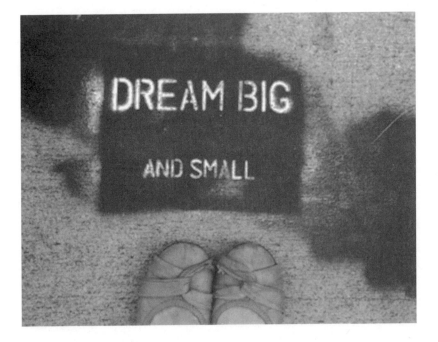

CHAPTER NINE

GREEN BEAUTY

"I don't want realism! I want magic! Yes, yes, *magic!*"
—Tennessee Williams (1911–1983),
American Author and Playwright, Survivor, Well-Dressed Bloke

Everyone in Los Angeles was beautiful. Every audition I went on, I was surrounded by younger, glowing, far more well-dressed versions of myself. The guys all looked like they stepped out of a catalogue for Malibu Ken and were trying to grab a latte *à la incognito*. Everyone seemingly knew how to look famous with ease. If I hadn't learned about sugar daddies before, I certainly did in LA! Just a few weeks after signing a modeling contract, I was getting all kinds of pressure I had never experienced before.

Boobs. *How were big boobs still a thing?* In New York City the smaller you were, the better. The less makeup you had on, the more likely you were to book a job. The more real you were, the bigger your paycheck.

But LA? If I went on five auditions in a day, I was instructed to dress five completely different ways. It was a standard expectation that I would get a blowout have my nails done, book weekly spa appointments, and treat myself to pedicures, massages, professional makeup artistry, and plastic surgery—all on the mere hope that this would land me jobs. It came with the field I had chosen, and I was extremely uncomfortable with all of it. As someone who had never even purchased a push-up bra, every single casting made me question if I was pursuing the right career.

Plus, I couldn't make friends with any of the girls I worked with. Without a sugar daddy, swanky Beverly Hills apartment, or wealthy celebrity uncle, every day I felt like I was swimming amongst a hungry swarm, blaring every SOS I could think of to stand out to casting directors, agencies, and brands.

When I wore my hair curly, they wanted it straight. When I blew my hair straight, someone *always* asked to see it curly. One week I was too skinny. The next month, when I managed to gain a few pounds, it "wasn't in the right places." This didn't seem like very constructive criticism to me. In a game that, for example, awarded major points to bring flowers on everyone's birthday, I was struggling to pay to travel to auditions. I barely remembered when my own birthday was . . .

I seemed to be losing at this particular game.

The Twenty-Five-Year-Old Virgin

However, I was surprised by how tiny of a town Hollywood really was, and how quickly I made it to parties among A-listers. I even auditioned for a feature movie and TV pilot within my first week in town. I found myself at private parties rooftop at The Standard, watching joints get passed around poolside in Santa Monica, and sipping miso soup at Katsuya with young Hollywood elite.

I popped into my new agency before a casting, and they said something that surprised me. The owner looked me over distastefully and demanded to know what products I was using on my skin. I had to admit the truth, if it wasn't totally obvious from my first six seconds of stammering. I wasn't really using *anything*. And I couldn't name anything off the top of my head either. I was a twenty-five-year-old beauty product virgin. In their eyes, I was perfectly hopeless.

They suggested I get a chemical peel. I nodded solemnly, portfolio in hand, my confidence sunk. On the way to my car I caught my reflection in a Mercedes window. Dry, bumpy, dehydrated skin. An acne-erupted jawline. Pockmarks. Early wrinkles. *Who was this girl staring back at me?*

That very day, determined to clean up my skin and win the heart of my agency, I furiously began researching the best of beauty, including the ingredients that made these products the best of the best.

Just one click, and I was horrified.

Beauty

An average of 75 percent of what we put on our skin gets absorbed into our bloodstream. That's what they say, but I'm willing to bet it's closer to 100 percent. After all, our skin is incredibly porous. It relies on us putting good things on it to stay youthful, hydrated, and to be optimally functional.

Our skin is the largest organ in our bodies.

There are over eight hundred chemicals in beauty products sold in the United States, many of which are potentially carcinogenic or harmful to the body in a variety of ways.

Do these two things seem a little incompatible to you?

The Greatest Beauty Myth

Sodium lauryl sulfate (SLS) and sodium laureth sulfate (SLES) are potentially the most harmful ingredients in personal care products, and it'll be hard for you *not* to find them in your beauty cabinets or even in many popular bath and shower products designed for kids. Industrial use of SLS and SLES include garage floor cleaners, engine degreasers, and car wash soaps. Conventional beauty product use includes shampoos, conditioners, lathering soap, and bodywash. Large amounts of carcinogenic nitrates may enter the body in just one lather in the shower when we're dealing with shampoos, conditioners, or bodywashes that are made with SLS or SLES. Research has proven them both potentially carcinogenic.[16]

Some of the most common additives are substances like aluminum, often used in eye shadow or as a color additive. It's also in many deodorants. Aluminum is not only carcinogenic, it's toxic and a mutagen, meaning it *changes your cell structure*.[17]

Oxybenzone is another widely used ingredient. Often found in sunscreen, the last safety review of this product was done in the 1970s. A study done in 2008 revealed that 97 percent of Americans are contaminated with oxybenzone, and it's been linked to allergies, hormone disruption, and cell damage. This chemical is linked to low birth weight in baby girls whose mothers are exposed to it during pregnancy.[18]

Or take, for instance, BHA and BHT. These are preservatives used in moisturizers and makeup, which research has proven may cause cancer and are harmful to fish and other wildlife. BHT (butylated hydroxytoluene) is an antioxidant that slows down the rate at which products change color and has been banned in the EU because it's an immune system toxicant, endocrine disruptor, and probable human carcinogen.[19]

Parabens have finally gotten the recognition they've always deserved, and for all the wrong reasons. Parabens—methylparaben, propylparaben, isoparaben, and butylparaben—are a group of preservative chemicals that have been used in cosmetics and pharmaceuticals since at least the 1950s. About 85 percent of cosmetics contain parabens, and concerns have been raised because parabens display estrogenic activity, stimulating breast cancer. Even scarier? Any amount of paraben absorbed through the skin may be as high as ten times the concentration of an oral dose, making them especially toxic for beauty products! Twenty nanograms/gram of parabens have been detected in a small sample of twenty breast tumors. Methylparaben represents 62 percent of the parabens found in that study, in case you're wondering which parabens to really, *really* avoid.[20]

Then, there's mineral oil. Often considered a beneficial moisturizer, mineral oil is manufactured from crude oil. This is the number one chemical in cosmetics that leads to petrochemical hypersensitivity, causing allergic reactions, arthritis, migraines, epilepsy, and diabetes.[21] Petroleum is also a crude oil, and is found in petroleum jelly, and Vaseline products.

Trust

Did you rummage through your beauty cabinets and throw everything in the trash after looking at the labels? Stop! I'm not telling you these things to scare you, trust me. I say it because no matter how many mantras, how many affirmations, or how many exercises we do, we are at our happiest when our outside reflects the light we have inside.

Honestly, I was just as shocked as you were to examine many of my "natural" products and still find some of these ingredients. There seemed to be no way around them! Learning what they meant inspired about a week away from my beauty cabinet altogether. It's scary to learn that a lot of marketing has deceived us about what's good to put in and on our bodies. We can spend a lifetime reading about what's "The Best Foundation" or "The Best Way to Treat Acne" in glossy magazines, but turn some of these products around and you start to wonder why no one is talking about the harmful chemicals contained in each and every one of the things designed to promote beauty. Aisle after aisle. In store after store. I mean, it's madness!

This is the same reason why we have a hard time trusting our doctors when they themselves are out of shape, or trusting our parents when they aren't practicing what they're preaching to us. But our appearance can be the reason that we get a job, or don't. Have an opportunity, or miss one. You can tell right off the bat if someone is malnourished or well fed, happy or sad, aged or youthful. We want our outsides to match all the hard work we're doing on the inside. That's why it was especially difficult to live my life as a wellness coach and wellness warrior when my skin was breaking out like crazy.

I don't mean little breakouts either. Almost a year into my journey, after getting settled in my North Hollywood home, my skin was worse than it had ever been. I prayed for the breakouts I had back in New York when I had seen a dermatologist and decided not to take minocycline. Every day I woke up with bigger, more painful bumps on my face and body with absolutely no trace of a solution.

The Culprit

We've all had bad days when it comes to our skin. Between harsh smog, toxic chemicals in our body products, the environment, and day-to-day stress, it's hard to know what's causing all the dissatisfaction on our faces or bodies. I realized that even though I was treating my body very well from the inside, I definitely needed to do something on the outside to care for my skin and do my best to have the even, dewy, freckly-in-all-the-right-places complexion I always dreamed of having.

My battle was going to be an uphill one. About three months settled into Los Angeles, I was at my wit's end. Not only was my skin totally erupted in acne that looked kind of like boils, it was incredibly dry, painful, and every time I showered I always felt like I had a "film" over my body that no amount of washing could get off! *Was something wrong with me?*

Also, my hair felt like straw! In New York, I had grown out my mermaid curls with pride for years. Just before I moved they had reached the middle of my back. Long, dark, lovely locks were what I had spent years dreaming of, and it was so comforting to have mermaid hair that fell below my chest. All I had needed was a trim here and there in the homeland to keep them up.

But right after the New Year 2012 in Los Angeles, I was ready to shave my head. It made me cry daily.

First of all, my hair had turned naturally ombré (not cute ombré, *damaged* ombré) from the California sun and salt water, which were leaving my now straw-blond ends extremely dry. There were parts under my crown that were actually *starting to dread*, and not one single brand of conditioner, brushing, combing, or "natural" oil treatment was working to stop this crazy process. The breakage and damage went all the way to the roots, and I was upset because it looked downright silly to have kinky, dry hair I had no control over when I was preaching a healthy lifestyle.

I was also getting acne on my body, and it wasn't the occasional bacne I'm talking boils on my *hips*, cysts on my neck, and my legs started to break out in bouts of psoriasis, a skin condition I hadn't been face-to-face with since high school. My face got so dry I couldn't even hope to wear makeup. It didn't matter what moisturizer I used, it always stung and made the dryness worse.

Immediately, I confided in some girlfriends about what to do. My best friend in Hollywood, Jasmine, suggested that I get my hair "done" and speak to a stylist about what the causes and solutions might be. I booked an appointment right away.

That stylist had absolutely no idea what the problem could be, and tried to push expensive, chemical-laden products on me (a few of which I bought) to help solve it. It wasn't until a few weeks later, on a photo shoot, that the hair and makeup artist there told me she shaved her head *twice* after she moved to Los Angeles before she found the culprit:

Her own shower!

Who would have thought that my biggest skin enemy didn't lie in my food, my environment, my skin care routine, or my genes? My biggest skin enemy was just plain hard water! Hard water is water high in alkaline (high pH) that also contains high levels of magnesium, calcium, iron, or calcium ions, and many cities in the United States, including Los Angeles, are full of it. The "buildup" of these minerals makes it hard for other things, such as soaps or detergents, to dilute and dissolve, leaving a surface residue on your skin when you shower, or worse, take a bath, which I was doing a lot of. This clogs and irritates the skin, which explained everything from the filmy feeling on my body to my straw-like hair to my red, itchy skin to my psoriasis flare-ups. I had to laugh.

You'll know if you have hard water if you experience any of the symptoms of dry skin, itchiness, or a filminess right after showering. You can also easily research the hard water in your area at: www.theorganiclifeblog.com/hardwater

Soft Water

I immediately got myself a showerhead filter (the one I bought was from Culligan). For less than forty dollars I wondered what had ever stopped me from doing this before, *just in case*. The remedy for hard water is turning it back into soft water, which is water in its purest form. Soft water is important for regular hydration as well as for use on the skin and hair during showers and baths.

I also started to incorporate more filtered water into my diet. I would fill up a huge gallon jug of cold water from the showerhead and then add antioxidant fruits or veggies like lemons, blueberries, basil, mint, or cucumber. This discouraged me from avoiding drinking plain water because it "didn't taste good" (a favorite excuse of mine and one that runs in my family). Drinking just one glass of water in the morning straight out of bed can increase energy, productivity, and alertness.

Seventy percent of the human body is comprised of water, with muscles being made of 70 percent water as well as blood needing 80 percent water, so soft water plays an important part in our optimum function. A glass of water first thing in the morning has been proven to clear toxins, fight infections, and boost our body's metabolism.[22]

Take the time to place the water there before you sleep, so it's available throughout the night as needed. If nature calls in the middle of the night, answer! I started drinking a glass in the morning, every morning, before I even got out of bed, just because it was *right there*. If you don't feel like you have the time for this, set your alarm five minutes earlier. Drinking water before you eat anything actually has more benefits than those extra five minutes of sleep!

Drinking a glass of soft water in the morning all but cured my nausea, which fluctuated depending on my position in my wellness process. I was so ready for my withdrawal symptoms *to be over*, but I figured it might take at least a year if I'd been on most of the prescription drugs for over ten years. Some days were better than others, and I learned to accept this progress as the drawling teacher that it was.

I began to drink the recommended eight glasses of water a day, plus tons of cups of herbal, caffeine-free tea. It's very important to avoid caffeine while trying to clean up your skin, age well, and/or detoxify, because caffeine is a dehydrating appetite suppressant.

The other incredible thing about getting an inexpensive water filter was that good, clean, filtered water was now completely free. This magical substance, which continued to help me battle my bladder infections, cleanse my blood, boost my immunity, clear my skin, and cure my nausea didn't cost me a thing. And if I threw some fresh lemon, cucumber, mint, or berries in the mix, I also had a great-tasting, Pinterest-worthy beverage all day long.

Many of us just plain forget how great water is for us. How integral it is to our health and our system functioning. We've been sold so many energy drinks, fast, carbonated, chemical-laden beverages, and sugar water disguised as "juice" that sometimes, pure water is the one thing left that we can really trust. I started to think of water as an essential nutrient, like a meal, that I needed to keep my body going.

It totally worked.

Your Skin's Worst Enemy

Coffee, the beverage many of us rely on completely to wake up, get work done, or succeed, may be causing us to age and experience a dull complexion much more than we think. Caffeine, the additive that gives us the jolt in coffee, is a drug that's been known to cause anxiety, insomnia, nervousness, upset stomach, restlessness, and liver spots, and it wreaks havoc on our skin.

Caffeine is extremely dehydrating because it's a diuretic. It's also extremely addictive, which is why headaches, irritability, and mood swings are common among those who try to stop drinking coffee.

Herbal teas are pretty much the opposite of coffee, and they were my solution to replacing a habit of drinking adult beverages by noon with a healthy alternative. In fact, many herbal teas can have similar effects and even a similar taste to coffee if blended right for energy, vitality, and concentration. Better yet, there's no crash!

My favorite herbal teas are the ones you make yourself from dried or picked herbs, but my favorite brands are Yogi Tea, Buddha Teas, Kusmi Tea, and Teeccino (these are coffee-like herbal teas that are perfect for anyone trying to come off coffee!).

My Face

Now that my hard-water problem was solved, I was dead set on fixing up my face! I researched *dermatitis*, which the hard water had really irritated around my chin, jawline, and mouth. Dermatitis is a general term for hard, red bumps that appear on the face, and are most common in women in their mid-twenties to early forties. Dermatitis is inflammation of the skin that can cause small, hard bumps that are almost impossible to treat. They can be caused by everything from clothing irritants, to sodium laureth sulfates or parabens, to genetics. One of the first brands that came up in my search of products for dermatitis was Osmia Organics.

Our Faces

Let me start by saying that all Osmia Organics products are natural, organic, and they didn't break my bank like many other acne products I had used. What can be better than that? Not only did the brand owner, Dr. Sarah Villafranco, suffer from perioral dermatitis herself, but her story also sounded a lot like mine. After years of trying product after product to soothe her skin, Sarah began developing natural products of her own. Oh, so it wasn't just me who suffered from a serious case of "What the hell is up with my face?"

Sarah makes a black clay facial soap with black Australian clay and Dead Sea mud that claimed to balance and tone the skin. It had incredible reviews on the Osmia website, from ladies suggesting it had completely cleared their acne, to women with no skin problems at all saying that it was great for cleansing and made their skin feel great. I immediately ordered some, and couldn't wait for my first package!

"Everything has beauty, but not everyone sees it."
—Confucius (551 BC–479 BC), Chinese Teacher,
Philosopher, Politician, Multi-Passionate Fellow

Love at First Sniff

With an olive oil base, palm kernel oil, mango, and sweet almond oil, I could smell this soap right through the package on my front stoop! Even though I hadn't used soap on my face in years because of its harsh, drying qualities, I lathered up at the sink and gave this Black Clay Facial Soap a try immediately!

Along with an assortment of other awesome full-size soap samples and a honey myrrh lip balm, the Black Clay Facial Soap came with a sweet note. It read:

> *Tara:*
> *Here are some soap samples and the Honey-Myrrh Lip Repair!*
> *Hope you enjoy, and good luck as you continue on your journey!*
> *—Best, Sarah*

I had never received a package with a personal note attached to it before, never mind one from the brand owner and creator herself! I fell in love with Osmia on a whole other level and felt more inspired than I had in years. I reached out to Sarah immediately and told her I would absolutely love to blog about my experience.

As far as healthy living was concerned, I didn't think there was anything worth writing about besides an experience or two with new raw-food places in Los Angeles. My experience with sobriety was so new, I wasn't sure what to even say about it. However, my experience with Osmia's products was enough for me to really want to start putting my opinion "out there."

I raved about the products in a post entitled "Tara Ogles Osmia Organics."[23] The post shows me using their lip repair and soap in my bathroom. It was cute and informative, but pretty amateurish. I knew I was creating something no one had really done before, and I wasn't sure where to start. So I did what I was most comfortable with; I was honest, I did my own photography with my own editing, and I recommended the post to a few female friends who I knew were suffering from troubled skin.

The Response

The response was overwhelmingly positive! All my girlfriends wanted to know if this soap was really working to cure my face and heal my acne, and I could honestly tell them that *it was*! After just a week of use I noticed absolutely remarkable results created by the combination of a good diet, along with DIM, supplements, omegas, fish oil, and this incredible new soap! It couldn't be denied. When I saw my girlfriends, they commented about how much better my skin looked. I was still well on my way to "perfect," but my friends were intrigued! After seeing how much clearer my skin looked, they were all curious where they too could find all-natural, non-irritating brands to heal their complexions.

Eager to discover more organic beauty products, I turned to the Internet once again for more brands to try, but I was very surprised to find that there weren't very many blogs focusing on green, healthy, organic products to use for better skin, and ultimately, a better life.

So I started my own blog, which I called *My Organic Life*. My journey to an all-green life was finally coming together, and I was ready to share my journey—all of it—with the world.

Clays for Health

The first record of medicinal clay goes back to Mesopotamia. Mud therapy is common among spas, but not exactly encouraged for us all to use in our day-to-day lives. There are different clays for different kinds of skin.

Ask yourself:

What type of skin do I have?

OILY SKIN:

Clogged pores, shiny, thick complexion, enlarged pores, constant severe acne, post-blemish red/dark scars that linger, acne-prone or oily-feeling skin.

DRY SKIN:

Almost invisible pores, dull, rough complexion, red patches, less elasticity, visible lines, flaky feeling. Prone to aging and wrinkles.

NORMAL SKIN:

No or few imperfections, no severe sensitivity, barely visible pores, radiant complexion. (The rest of us envy you, by the way.)

COMBINATION SKIN:

Overly dilated pores, blackheads, shiny skin. Patches of dry and oily skin.

SENSITIVE SKIN:

Sensitive skin is usually dry, feels tight, and becomes inflamed and irritated easily. Typically, sensitive skin develops red or scaly areas, can be itchy and tingly, and is prone to breakouts.

TROUBLED SKIN:

As mentioned, I'd always had pretty troubled skin. I had combination skin that was sun damaged and very acne prone. Even while I was on birth control it had never been perfect, but I'd really never had to give it a second thought. However, this new bout of breakouts was something else! I was so desperate to fix it, and I didn't have to research very long before coming across my very first solution. . . .

FRENCH GREEN CLAY

French green clay was my first clay savior. I bought it in bulk of one pound, which lasted me almost *two years*, even though I used it every single day in some way, shape, or form once I first bought it. French green clay is marvelous for helping to clear problem skin, making your own skin-clearing concoctions, fixing up troubled spots, or just for weekly gentle use by itself for antiaging. Combined with other clays, it's a total powerhouse!

Depending on the purity of the green clay it works as an aggressive absorbent to soak up all the oil and toxicity that is causing clogged pores and breakouts in your skin.

The Self-Love Beauty Ritual

Step 1: Take a tablespoon of French green clay and place it in your favorite bowl.

Step 2: Take an equal tablespoon of water and mix the two gently. If you need to add more clay, go for it! The consistency should be a little thick, not watery.

Step 3: Apply to problem areas: acne flare-ups, under-the-skin breakouts, acne scars, oily spots, dark circles, or your T-zone. It's perfectly safe to apply on the face or anywhere on the body! But avoid the mouth because, while it's natural, it doesn't taste very good!

> **Step 4:** Let it dry. Go take a bath, answer emails, do some stretches. It should take about ten to fifteen minutes to dry completely.
> **Step 5:** Wash it off with filtered warm water. Pat your beautiful face dry. Rinse with cold water.
> **Step 6:** Follow with a glass of cold water. As mentioned, clays are dehydrating!

French green clay literally "drinks up" your skin's bad oils, so you will know when you're ready to wash this—or any—clay mask off *right before* it becomes hard like cracked mud. Don't let it sit on your face long once it's completely dry, as you'll be letting the crap it just soaked up sit atop your skin too!

Apply, let it dry, and rinse it off.

That was all there was to it, and I immediately saw results. It zapped the oil from my skin, and my complexion became clearer *the very next day*! This is not an exaggeration, and a large part of the reason I am so passionate about clay masks for getting and maintaining healthy skin. I was finally seeing the results of "zapping" the infected area that had eluded me when using everything from Proactiv to probiotics! *Finally!*

If that's all there is to it, then *why didn't I know about it before? Why doesn't everyone do it to clear their skin and prevent signs of aging?* I wasn't positive how to answer that myself. I had used a "hydrating" mask or two in my day, but clay masks were a totally new (but very intuitive) concept to me.

FULLER'S EARTH

Let's face it, no matter how effective the products you put all over your face to control your breakouts may be, sometimes you *need* to target specific spots, blemishes, and imperfections without smearing something all over yourself. This is where fuller's earth comes in.

Fuller's earth has been used as a "skin lightening" agent for years. Some darker-skinned mixed girls I knew had used it to "bleach" their skin (back in the day, when being pale was cooler than being tan). Being the palest mixed girl I knew, this was not my interest. I wanted to use it as a spot treatment—on scars.

It's great for red skin, or skin prone to acne, or complexions with overactive oil production. Like French green clay, fuller's earth literally draws oils and toxins out of the skin, and is used industrially as an agent for many skin care products for this exact reason.

Fuller's earth was great for my acne scars! I was making real progress and only had scars left instead of bumps I had to fight all the time, so this clay became my new best friend! I only used it for spot treatments, so a pound of it lasted me over a year.

The Goddess Ritual

Step 1: Take a tablespoon of fuller's earth clay and place it in your favorite bowl.

Step 2: Take an equal tablespoon of water, rose water, and/or aloe and mix the ingredients gently until you reach a muddy texture.

Step 3: Apply to problem areas with a fan brush or clean fingers. The face or anywhere on the body is perfectly safe. It is safe to ingest if it happens accidentally, but I wouldn't recommend it.

Normally when a wound from picking my face had finally clotted and healed and the new skin naturally fell off, it would always have revealed a pick mark, a scar, or just simply start bleeding again! But this daily spot treatment was miraculous! It would literally "peel" my skin. This means that if I had an active breakout that had turned into a clot with a dry-skin barrier, the barrier would fall off and reveal new, beautiful, youthful skin when I washed my face mask off instead of a scar! I was totally amazed. This *sold me* completely on clays.

BENTONITE CLAY

A ton of minerals are found in bentonite clay. This clay *will* lift oil, toxins, radioactive chemicals, or heavy metals out of your skin, and it's great for accelerated healing and nourishment. It contains over fifty minerals, and is totally natural. It can be used as a clay mask as well as a spot treatment on the face and body for acne, acne scars, and flare-ups. When ingested it can do wonders for your digestion as well.

Yep, that's right. I said you should eat it.

CLAY SMOOTHIES

Have you ever seen your pet eat dirt and said, "Oh my gosh, Fluffy! Not again!"?

Fluffy's actually eating clay, and she's pretty intuitive (and probably going to poop soon). She instinctively knows that clay really helps with digestion. So, how come Fluffy knows this, but I had no idea until I was two and a half decades old?

I honestly can't answer that question, but I'm sure at some point I inherited the desire to want to eat dirt from my ancestors. I'm pretty positive human beings used to eat *a lot* of dirt between eating sour meat hanging from a cave wall and waiting for the crops to grow.

So with Fluffy and my ancestors serving as an example, I also added a teaspoon of bentonite clay into my smoothies in the morning, in addition to using it on my face as a mask. I couldn't even taste it, and it was very detoxifying!

The Clay Detox Smoothie

Step 1: Combine a tablespoon of bentonite clay with some cucumber, celery, water, ginger, and mint in a blender.
Step 2: Blend the tonic on high.
Step 3: Drink up! This is going to work lovingly on your liver, colon, tummy, and your entire bloodstream, and it will help your body process toxins and other foods.

Unfired clay is a vital reactive substance known as "living earth." Bentonite clay has an electrical charge, so when it comes in contact with a toxin, it will absorb the little bugger, which makes it great for masks and cleansing.

The reason I put it in my smoothies is because drinking bentonite before bed at night and first thing in the morning is the best way to make sure that it won't come in contact with any other metals you may ingest throughout the day. This is so important, because other metals and ions can interfere with its ability to naturally help you!

Once again, drink PLENTY of water! I cannot overstate this enough! Clay is very dehydrating to the skin and body, but that is because it is drawing out all the unwanted toxins and bad metals in your body! It also cleanses the colon, promotes digestion, and increases T-cells and oxygen in the bloodstream.

The Cleansing Mineral Ritual

Step 1: Place a teaspoon of bentonite clay into an eight-ounce glass of cold water. Use a wooden spoon if you can to avoid metal interference.
Step 2: If you use a metal spoon, immediately remove the metallic spoon from the glass.

Step 3: Let it sit for however long you can. Half an hour to overnight is recommended.

Step 4: Drink up! Sip it throughout your day, or do multiple glasses! If you really can't stand the taste, throw it in a smoothie as mentioned.

CLAY WRAPS & GANDHI'S INFLUENCE

Clay wraps were the next logical step in my process, and stemmed from combating psoriasis and those strange cystic breakouts on my hips, elbows, arms, and legs. I would "wrap" them in wet clay and gauze overnight, and was consistently surprised by the incredible outcome. My redness and irritation diminished and then vanished completely, my breakouts were less frequent and clearing up, and as an extra bonus my stretch marks were disappearing! The results really just couldn't be denied.

I also used to wrap my stomach in bentonite clay with gauze when I was very nauseous and it worked miracles! I first read about this in Gandhi's autobiography *The Story of My Experiments with Truth*, in which he swears by clay wraps for digestion and toxic ailments. He even used clay wraps to treat the bubonic plague (all of Gandhi's patients treated with this method *survived* the black plague, while every other patient treated in the same hospital with conventional methods died!).

Be sure to hydrate a lot when you do this, because the clay is essentially pulling the toxins out around your organs. In rare cases, you may get nauseous or sick, in which case, allow yourself to do so. And keep hydrated! Although we have a great stigma to vomiting in this country, it's entirely healthy for your body to purge toxins if you are doing a cleansing. There is nothing wrong with throwing up. It's completely natural if you are not forcing it; it's your body's way of communicating to you.

ACTIVATED CHARCOAL

Okay, okay . . . this one isn't exactly a clay. But I've thrown at least a little bit of activated charcoal into every clay mask I've ever made, and it was the most active ingredient of the first clay soap I used, so it's worth a good, long mention.

Activated charcoal, also known as activated carbon, has been a godsend for clearing and cleaning up my skin, promoting youthfulness, and aiding in my digestion. It's been used for thousands of years all over the world because it draws bacteria, dirt, poisons, chemicals, and other nasty microparticles from the body in a safe and natural way. Activated charcoal has been proven to absorb one hundred to two hundred times its weight in impurities, making it a deep-cleansing agent.[24] The same treatments that cost up to $400 at some spas can be done at home with some French green clay and a capsule or two of activated charcoal *for less than a dollar*, which can also be taken internally to detoxify, treat poison, treat GI-tract infections, help withdrawals, and aid in curing nausea.

It can be used to whiten the teeth as well! Add a dash of activated charcoal to your toothpaste on your brush twice a day for instant results!

The Devotee's Detox Ritual

Step 1: Prepare a clay base (French green clay or bentonite both work great) by adding one tablespoon to your favorite bowl.

Step 2: Add one tablespoon of activated charcoal to the clay.

Step 3: Mix with a tablespoon of purified water, or organic aloe water.

Step 4: Spread lovingly on your face with a fan brush or your fingers.

Step 5: Allow it to dry and work its magic for ten to fifteen minutes. Make a cup of tea, read a chapter of a book, make a gratitude list, create a playlist, and relax.

Step 6: Wash it off with warm water followed by cleansing your face with cold water.

Incorporating activated charcoal into your daily skin care ritual will leave you with a calmer, clearer complexion. It has been a total lifesaver for maintaining my skin. Whenever I am at a point where my skin has become totally unmanageable, I will do this mask and ingest a 500-mg capsule of activated charcoal internally. I also add a dash of activated charcoal (anywhere from a pinch to a table-spoon) into my blender in the morning and it clears it right up!

It's great for soothing the effects of pharmaceutical withdrawal, which I was most definitely still experiencing when I started using it, and it works wonders as a regular everyday detox and for health promotion.

RHASSOUL CLAY

Moroccan Rhassoul clay is naturally found in the Atlas Mountains in northeastern Morocco. It's been used by Roman and Egyptian nobility as a beauty agent, and is wonderful for toning up your complexion.

Rhassoul clay is extraordinarily mineral-rich, highly absorbent, and contains a high rate of ion exchange and provitamins that are instantly absorbed into and used by the skin when applied. Clinical testing has shown it to improve skin elasticity, unclog pores, and remove surface oils and dead skin cells. It can also be used on the scalp as a hair mask or a dry shampoo for absorbing excess oils.

For me, Rhassoul clay worked on days where nothing else truly did. I'd do my overnight charcoal masks, but some days my skin was just so damn bumpy, infected, red, and puffy that it felt like nothing would drain it of all the gunk. My skin felt absolutely poisoned, and I was hopeless, afraid to look in the mirror, afraid to touch my face, afraid to look at myself naked in case I had another breakout somewhere new.

Rhassoul clay *did the job*, hands down. Not only did it improve my skin, fight acne, and lighten acne scars, it dried up stubborn pimples that just wouldn't go away for weeks.

If you have drier and sensitive skin, you may want to wear your Rhassoul clay mask for a shorter amount of time, but the normal ten to fifteen minutes with the preparation mentioned in the Devotee's Daily Ritual will clear away your most stubborn blemishes in no time if you have particularly troubled skin.

KAOLIN CLAY

Kaolin clay made its way into my life when a company sent me samples to review on my blog. Kaolin is an incredible clay made from the soils that have been weathered from a hot, moist climate, like the tropical rain forest. It's named after the hill in China where it was mined for centuries, Kao-Ling. Kaolin clay is incredibly nourishing to the skin, and some even claim that kaolin is hydrating, despite being a clay! It works by removing the excess amount of sebum—the oil that the skin produces—which can clog pores if left untreated.

While this clay is a super effective clay mask—and one of my favorites—it is also good for warding off radiation if you ingest a little bit of kaolin with your daily food intake. Another favorite cleansing ritual of mine is throwing a pinch or two of kaolin clay into my baths at night for some extra detox action!

The Beauty Bath Ritual

Step 1: Draw a hot bath.
Step 2: While you wait for it to cool, add in your favorite essential oils, plants, flower petals, or salts.
Step 3: Add three tablespoons of kaolin clay. Mix lovingly with your hands or a wooden spoon.
Step 4: Let the clay absorb for ten minutes and allow the bathwater to cool down. Slip in with your favorite book and let your body detoxify in your clay-infused spa water! Practice your favorite meditations, affirmations, or breathing exercises. *Relax.*
Step 5: Follow with many glasses of ice water.

OILS

Using oil for my breakouts initially seemed counterintuitive to me. *So I'm going to put oil onto something that's infected with excess oil? How will that help?*

Balance, my friends. It turns out that finding the correct oil to balance your skin can create miraculous overnight benefits! Not all oil is evil, and not all oils are created equal!

Basically, the oil that your face produces is mostly fatty acids that your skin actually *needs* to stay properly hydrated and sexy. The oil acts as the skin's lipid barrier and protects against extreme temperatures, dryness, or over-cleansing.

Cream moisturizers and balms are mostly water-based. Oils, however, contain no added water and are a much more powerful way to deliver all of the nutrients you need deep into your skin for proper balance and hydration.

GOLDEN JOJOBA

The first time I had heard of jojoba was in college, when I wrote an entire thesis about its uses as a natural gas for vehicles. I never thought I'd be putting it on my skin!

Jojoba oil (pronounced *ho-ho-ba*) isn't actually oil at all; it's closer to sebum, the oil your body naturally pumps out when it's dehydrated. Jojoba oil is classified as a liquid wax, and it can do everything from balance your skin to power your car! The wax is distilled from the seeds of the jojoba plant, which are mostly grown in North America. In the 2002 book *Jojoba: New Crop for Arid Lands, New Raw Material for Industry*, the National Research Council notes that acne treatments containing jojoba oil slow the outbreak of skin breakouts caused by acne.

Because of its close relation to our natural skin sebum, jojoba oil is absorbed easily and readily into the skin. It's gentle, softening, and can be used to stimulate hair growth (such as on the eyebrows or scalp). It's also an effective makeup remover and facial cleanser all on its own!

Jojoba oil was one of the first natural oils that I purchased in bulk for my skin, and boy did it work wonders! For me, jojoba oil was the answer I had always been looking for. It created a glowing, golden complexion. My skin loved it—I could accidentally overuse some and it wouldn't cause a single adverse reaction. My big, thirsty pores drank it up and shrugged off the excess. No clogged pores, no oily residue, no funky smell (no smell at all, in fact!). It also made a great oil base for treating everything from a scratchy throat to a restless night's sleep; simply add a few drops of lavender and peppermint and rub on the affected area.

The Golden Goddess Ritual

Step 1: Clean hands with an all-natural cleanser, or the jojoba oil itself.

Step 2: Add a few drops of jojoba oil into your favorite bowl. You can add a few drops of your favorite face-friendly essential oils if you like (ylang-ylang, vitamin E, or neroli are good to start with). If you do this, inhale. This is a wonderful aromatherapy in itself!

Step 3: Use a cotton ball or clean fingers to gently rub the jojoba oil onto your cleansed face. Doing this slowly in circles toward your heart stimulates blood flow. Let sit for one to four minutes.

Step 4: Rinse with filtered warm water and a clean face towel. Pat dry. Cleanse with cold water.

COCONUT OIL

When I started incorporating oils into my skin care regimen, coconut oil was getting its first little bout of recent hype, but I was already on the bandwagon, hard. Coconut oil had been incredible for me once I scaled down and figured out how to use it.

At first, I slathered it on like a skin balm. I loved the way this oil smelled and felt so much that I couldn't help myself! My skin was not happy with that *at all*! Coconut oil is mostly saturated fats, which retain the moisture of the skin by getting under it. If your skin is severely dehydrated, you can see how this would be incredibly helpful! But, if your skin is also sensitive, or oily to start with, you can see how these fats might clog the pores, leading to more breakouts that are harder to treat.

I finally drew the line at half a teaspoon. That's about all my face could handle. My body can bathe in it, but my face only liked a little bit!

Learn how much of this lovely oil your body can *actually* handle. Your sense of smell may try to convince you otherwise, but apply a bit at a time and gradually increase the amount until you find what's perfect for you and your particular skin. If the intoxicating scent simply calls to you, you can also do as I did and add a few drops to your smoothies in the morning, or to your meals!

Coconut oil has thousands of different uses; it's a delicious cooking oil, an excellent makeup remover, a scrumptious Teeccino creamer, and it was doing amazing things for my skin, hair, and nails. It was a great lip moisturizer for the dry California heat, and it was balancing out the oil production on my body by helping my skin create a natural barrier that both protected and nurtured itself. Not only is coconut oil great smelling and sexy to use, it works wonders on sore muscles, even without any essential oils added.

Coconut Oil Massage Ritual

Step 1: Grab your favorite jar of natural, organic coconut oil and a wooden spoon.
Step 2: Scoop coconut oil gently into your favorite bowl.

> **Step 3:** Add your favorite essential oil: eucalyptus, menthol, and peppermint for a muscle relaxer, lavender for a calm feeling, ylang-ylang to attract beauty.
> **Step 4:** Rub on yourself or a partner's affected sore areas, or use lovingly as a massage. Repeat your favorite affirmation to yourself.

ARGAN OIL

The *New York Times* recently termed it, "liquid gold."[25] Argan oil is created by extracting the oil from argan tree nuts. Argan is found in Morocco, Algeria, and Israel, and so far, studies indicate uses ranging from treating prostate cancer to lowering cholesterol to healing and preventing aging in the skin.[26]

I recommend eating argan oil, either in your smoothies or juices, or cooking with it, along with applying it directly to your skin for maximum benefits. In Morocco, it's used to dip bread or as a drizzle on couscous or pasta.

Argan oil is a beautiful golden color and the natural smell is absolutely lovely. You don't have to ask me twice to put anything golden directly onto my skin!

As mentioned, I experienced a lot of hair loss after coming off birth control and while going through withdrawal. The back of my head was thinning out and not even switching to brushing more gently was helping. I did a bit of research, which suggested "stimulating" the hair follicles with hair masks, like coconut or olive oil. Since I was still looking for a healthy alternative to coconut oil for anything around my face, I purchased argan oil at Whole Foods and made a hair mask with it that very night.

Some dripped onto my face during my at-home process (which involved wrapping my head up in a towel). This had been my concern with using coconut oil, because my face didn't like it much, but I didn't think twice about doing it with argan oil. Instead, I rubbed it into my skin lovingly.

The Hot Hair Mask Ritual

Step 1: Pour a cup of argan oil or your favorite nourishing oil into a pan.

Step 2: Heat pan over low heat on the stove until the oil is warm, but not too hot or sizzling.

Step 3: Transfer the warm oil into your favorite bowl.

Step 4: Brush warm oil through your hair gently with your preferred hairbrush, focusing on roots and ends.

Step 5: Put your hair up in a bun, then wrap with a shower cap or towel.

Step 6: Relax. Let the oils soak in for as long as you desire; overnight is best!

Step 7: Rinse with warm, filtered water.

Treating your hair with argan oil will promote shine, nourish your hair, help restore split ends, lubricate scalp dryness, and protect the skin and hair from future damage.

MARULA OIL

Marula oil is an all-natural, cold-pressed, highly nutritious light and exotic fruit seed oil made from the kernels of the drought-resistant, super durable Marula trees that are indigenous to southern Africa and Madagascar. I was first introduced to Marula oil when a company called African Botanics, who use it in the majority of their products, reached out to me through my blog.

This healing oil is widely used throughout South Africa for medicinal purposes, and has been a part of beauty rituals for both men and women for centuries. It has high concentrations of nutrients, antioxidants (including vitamin C and vitamin E), minerals, and fatty acids (like omegas 9 and 6, and monounsaturated fats, which our bodies love!) that repair and hydrate the deepest levels of the skin. Marula oil is great for use on the face as well as the body. The strong antimicrobial and antibacterial properties mean it needs no preservatives to last you a significant amount of time!

Not only is Marula oil great for the skin, its production is actually beneficial to various southern African communities. African Botanics' oil is sourced through a fair-trade program, and for this reason, I was all about it!

Marula oil was like jojoba oil on steroids for my skin! On top of my jojoba oil cleansing, I applied Marula oil to my face and body every night, every morning, and after every shower.

The Good Energy Ritual

Step 1: Shake a few drops of Marula oil onto your palms.

Step 2: Rub your palms together fast enough to create friction. Say a loving mantra to yourself, such as, "I am strong and beautiful."

Step 3: Pat the oil around your face, then use your hands to rub it gently in circles toward your heart to stimulate blood flow, circulation, and good energy.

By indulging in this short little ritual, you will experience a loving, caring sense of self, and a supported connectedness to your inner beauty. When love for yourself fully runs the show, the journey in beauty really begins!

BARBARY FIG SEED OIL

About a year after I started my blog, I heard about Barbary fig seed oil (sometimes called prickly pear oil) through a company called La Bella Figura. This company was all over the green-beauty community on Instagram, and was receiving a lot of attention from beauty mavens and bloggers.

Pure, raw, organic Barbary fig seed oil contains exceptionally high doses of vitamin E and vitamin K, linoleic acid, and betalains, which protect against free radicals, stimulate new cell growth, and hydrate the face, body, and nails.

The lovely founders of La Bella Figura were the fabulous women who brought Barbary fig seed oil to the West, and I will forever give them credit for turning me on to this gem.

After years of stress, anxiety, drugs, sleep deprivation, alcohol, and a toxic city environment, the bags under my eyes (yep, the same ones that were down to my cheekbones by the age of ten) were turning into serious milia, where the dry spots under the eyes morph into perma-bumps in your twenties.

No other product had ever delivered an instant glow (I mean immediately!), but Barbary fig seed oil instantly gave me smooth, fresh-looking skin! I swear even when I had breakouts, the oil was doing its best to "cover" them with its dewy, refreshing goodness.

This precious oil is highly rejuvenating to the skin. It slows down the aging of skin cells immediately, producing overnight results. Its benefits are three to four times greater than those of argan oil, clinically. Prickly pear's been proven to eliminate wrinkles, help even out skin, and treat hyperpigmentation.[27] And if you have cute little freckles that you're especially fond of, rest assured that it won't affect their pigmentation—at least it didn't for me. In fact, it brought out the attractive ones while nourishing dehydrated places, like the bags under my eyes. Prickly pear seed oil quickly became my skin superfood.

The Antiaging Oil Ritual

Step 1: Shake a few drops of organic Barbary fig seed oil onto your palms.

Step 2: Rub your palms together fast enough to create friction. Say something loving to yourself, such as, "I am vibrant!"

Step 3: Pat the oil around your face, concentrating on under your eyes and on your forehead. Use your fingertips to rub it gently in circles toward your heart to stimulate blood flow, circulation, and good energy.

VITAMIN E OIL

I first heard the true benefits of vitamin E oil through researching Waxelene, a company I had found through my newfound interest in organic, pesticide-free beeswax, which was the base of their product. Waxelene was also helpful for those impossible-to-treat dry patches on my skin, and in my garden. It helped protect the base of my plants against pests, and my hands became softer after a few weeks of using it. I had learned that Vaseline, a product I had slathered on everywhere from my eyelids to my toes, was full of highly toxic chemicals. Petroleum jelly was—shocker—made from petroleum! Petroleum jelly is made with crude oil, which can be toxic and harmful to the skin and system. Crude. Oil. *Ugh!*

Everything I used to use Vaseline for, I just used Waxelene for instead! It was super cheap, and Waxelene had only four ingredients, GMO-free organic soy oil, organic beeswax, natural vitamin E oil, and organic rosemary oil, and was touted all over the web as a great alternative to Vaseline. Everyone from Halle Berry's makeup artist to local mommy bloggers loved it.

The Waxelene helped with everything from household chores to hair masks, and the vitamin E intrigued me. Research has shown that vitamin E has strong antiaging and antioxidizing qualities, and promotes skin, hair, and nail growth. It's easily absorbed into the skin, both as a supplement or a beauty product, and you don't need a ton of it for it to be effective. Vitamin E impacts skin function on a cellular level, and the consumption of vitamin E has remarkable curative powers, from healing wounds (like acne scars, psoriasis, or any dry skin you are currently battling) to fighting gout to aiding in recovery from chemotherapy to increasing hair growth. It helps cure fading scars swiftly, something I was desperately seeking.[28]

Even weeks after my breakouts stopped, I was still looking at skin that was totally destroyed from months of dehydration, picking, scarring, withdrawal—skin that had suffered greatly due to a past of drugs, partying, and straight-up neglect. It seemed as though nothing would make me look normal, or please, oh please, reverse all this damage that I had done before I knew better. It felt totally hopeless. I cried about my skin, I was scared to look in the mirror, I canceled important meetings with important people, I put my career on hold. I was so, so sad that my progress wasn't being reflected in my skin.

These scars stressed me out, and I broke out more. This endless cycle had to be stopped, so I took one last step: I upped my dosage of vitamin E to 200 mg. I also threw a drop into everything from my aromatherapy to my morning bath oil.

I truly saw improvements in my scars overnight. Eventually, I stressed about my skin less, I worried less, I broke out less, I felt more like myself, and the amazing cycle continued!

Do I still break out? Every once in a while I get very manageable small zits, but only when I forget my supplements and neglect my beauty rituals!

Toners

My battle didn't end with clays and oils. There was still one crucial step between clay masks and moisturizing; its name was toning.

Despite being clean and clear, my skin looked kind of rough. Just a few weeks in the California sun had done a little number on my pores, and I was forming wrinkles. I wasn't a big fan of SPF at the time (this too has its own round of scary chemicals), and I knew there was a reason my skin felt dull instead of radiant after all the hard work I was doing.

Your skin has an acid mantle made up of sweat and oil that you naturally produce, which gets stripped away when we use a cleanser, mask, or scrub, changing our organic pH balance. Although a little oil is a good thing, if you have troubled or oily skin, a toner can be the added acid that helps prevent bacterial buildup and keeps your skin in check.

STORE-BOUGHT CRAP

I wasn't sold on toners because every single one I had used in the past was alcohol-based and left my skin dry and irritated. That's because I was using harsh astringents, laden with parabens and chemicals that irritate the skin.

Natural toners work to restore this precious pH balance and keep skin hydrated, promoting balance. Toners that truly do the job work to lock in moisture—the moisture in the toner and the moisture in whatever oils or creams you use after the toner on your most precious and largest organ, your skin. They don't dry out your skin even more, which is how the store-bought ones I had used forever essentially work.

PLANT-BASED TONERS

"Drinking water is essential, but that water has to go through all of your other organs before getting to your skin." Josh Rosebrook, of the all-natural and organic Josh Rosebrook Skin and Hair Care line, explained this concept to me the first time we met in Los Angeles. It all finally made sense. Why not give your skin the added benefit and extra moisture so that it can lock in the moisture of other products you use? I was sold on the idea of toner that day.

Much like oils, not all toners are created equal. Josh's Hydrating Accelerator, for instance, is plant-based. The base water is organic infused aloe water, with organic oils of sunflower, coconut, grape seed, and almond, and herbal infusions of bilberry, neem oil, and skullcap, along with vitamins E, A, C, and B2. That's what I was talking about!

The Hydrating Accelerator isn't the only toner out there that I was psyched to try! Different toners infused with magic skin-healing oils from a few green beauty brands, including LBF, Gressa Skin, Delizioso Skincare, among others, were all quickly filling up my bathroom cabinet.

Toning can have overnight or immediate results, like it did for me. This is the last step in the process to clear your face *and keep it clear*! If you're willing to experiment with even some of the skin care methods suggested in this book, I commend you! It's really, *really* hard to switch over to green beauty products, especially when we haven't seen any results yet. Personally, I didn't have anything to lose; I figured that since nothing had worked before, and that everything else I used had been total crap, green beauty products were worth a shot, especially at affordable prices!

Toning is now one of my favorite rituals. It's refreshing, exuberating, and always feels loving and lovely. It brightens, tones, and keeps my skin looking and feeling soft and younger.

The Skin Cleansing Ritual

Step 1: Grab your favorite all-natural, plant-based toner.
Step 2: Wash your hands so you don't transfer any bacteria to your face or your product. Wet your skin with warm, filtered water to open your pores.
Step 3: Using a cotton ball or beauty sponge, apply the toner to the skin, focusing on problem areas and always working toward the heart.
Step 4: Breathe deeply and say softly, "I am protecting my skin and loving myself."
Step 5: Let the toner sit for a few minutes. Apply your favorite oil or moisturizer.

By doing this, you restore your skin to its natural pH, cleanse your skin of extra microbacteria, and even out your complexion.

Salts

Last, but certainly not least, I wanted to make sure that each and every bath that I took was really helping my pain and nourishing my body. As I mentioned in previous chapters, soaking in various types of salts was a crucial part of my recovery. Relaxing in warm water for a few minutes to a few hours can truly work miracles for your achy and sore muscles. They're also wonderfully relaxing, soothing, and comforting.

Pain Relief Soak Ritual

Step 1: Add your favorite Epsom salt and eucalyptus or peppermint oil to a hot bath.

Step 2: Relax. Get to your blank slate. Fall away.

Step 3: Say this loving sentence: "I am well, I am relaxed, I am flexible."

Step 4: Run cold water over yourself at "hot" intervals, making sure you remain at a good core body temperature.

Step 5: Repeat: "I am well. I am relaxed. I am flexible."

Step 6: When you open your eyes and emerge from the bath, drink plenty of cold water to rehydrate.

Staying Green

Discovering green beauty products has been one of the most rewarding parts of my journey to full recovery. I am constantly in awe of the new products and beautiful formulations currently available to help my skin heal and regenerate. I've even had a chance to collaborate with some of my favorite brands, with some of my favorite ingredients, and create my own natural, organic beauty products. My little bit of research turned into a full-length, beautiful story of synchronicity and magic. I'll touch on that later.

Beauty is all around us, and nature truly has so much to offer when it comes to healing from the inside out. Don't be afraid to try the natural products that Mother Earth has provided. We should always be willing to do more, be more, and accept more healthy alternatives into our daily routines.

Half the battle of looking beautiful is *feeling beautiful*. You don't have to compromise to look and feel your best.

Whole Beauty

The takeaway here is that all the little changes you make to your daily antiaging and skin care rituals matter. It's easy to forget to wash your face at night or to take your vitamins or supplements, but it's just as easy to spend an extra five minutes before bed to do so. When I don't neglect myself, my skin is dewy, freckly, golden, and even-toned, which I had only just dreamed about *months prior*! These small but terribly crucial antiaging and skin care rituals took me on one of the most incredible journeys of my life. I *fell in love* with skin care.

When you invest in yourself, *you* can really reap what you've spent weeks, months, or years sowing. You'll see that inner light become an outer glow. Once you start, you won't be able to stop, and once you start to truly understand all the benefits that Mother Nature has to offer, you will see results. You can become one with nature, work with it, and become truly cured by it. One ritual, one self-affirming, self-loving devotion to yourself at a time.

Skin care is exciting for me. It feels like a gift to myself, each and every time I take the time to focus on my skin. It may seem tedious at first and you may not see results at the snap of a finger, but your body and skin will thank you. And trust me, your seventy-year-old self will thank present-day you as well.

Natural Green Products on the Market That Contain the Clays and Oils Mentioned in This Chapter

French green clay: Acure Organics Cell Stimulating Facial Mask, Meow Meow Tweet's Deodorant Cream, and W3ll People's Mineral Setting Powder.

Fuller's earth: Osmia Organics Detox Exfoliating Mask and May Lindstrom Skin's The Problem Solver Mask.

Bentonite clay: Level Naturals Mud Bath Bomb and Aztec Secret Indian Healing Clay.

Activated charcoal: Soapwalla's Activated Charcoal and Petitgrain Soap Bar, La Bella Figura's Purifying Face Mask, and the One Love Organics heart-shaped cleansing sponge.

Rhassoul clay: Root Science Reborn mask, Gressa Skin's Dirty Pretty Things mask, and La Bella Figura's Bioactive Purifying Mask.

Kaolin clay: Aquarian Bath's Rose Clay, Acure Organics Argan Stem + CoQ10 Dry Shampoo, and La Bella Figura's crème blush.

Jojoba oil: Leahlani Skincare's Siren Serum, Gressa Skin's Balancing Cleanser, and Delizioso Skincare's TARA California Bronzing Mousse.

Coconut oil: Skinny's Coconut Oil, Leahlani Skincare's Coconut Infusion, and RMS Beauty's "Un" Cover-up concealer.

Argan oil: Acure Organics Coconut Argan Oil, Misoves Pure Balance Face Oil, and Lina Hanson's Face Serum.

Barbary fig seed oil: Mun's Akanari Brightening Youth Serum, Kahina's Prickly Pear Seed Oil, and Delizioso Skincare's TARA Radiant Glow Body Oil.

CHAPTER TEN

THE TEACHER APPEARS

"If you don't invite God to be your summer guest,
He won't appear in the winter of your life."
—Lahiri Mahasaya (1828–1895), Indian Yogi,
Loving Husband and Father, Sent to
"Reintroduce the Lost Practice of Yoga to the West"

The six months after Dad's initial cancer diagnosis came and went. I was so, so hopeful. Although they had sent his test results to every specialty lab in America, no one could determine exactly what kind of cancer he had. Every lab was stumped.

We were puzzled and disheartened when the diagnosis came back as stage IV, "rare, unknown," and Dad was put on an aggressive and expensive oral renal cell chemotherapy that was taken at home.

I visited often. During the summer my cousin commented, "I see you more now than when you lived here!" It was true, and it didn't stop. I took a plane to New York every month after I left for the first year, then every six weeks after. It was getting kind of ridiculous, but I always made enough money when I was in New York to justify it (even though I barely came home with any of it). Really, I just wanted to spend time with my family. The chemotherapy was not treating Dad well.

Therapy

In the first few months of taking the chemo, Dad had gotten very ashy, and his hair had turned completely white. His head seemed to even be a different shape! His energy was gone and his smile was forced, but his only complaint was that he couldn't taste his food. Dad's oncologist often let him "come off" the chemotherapy for the holidays, and was super impressed with his progress. I could tell that the doctor was very surprised that my dad was standing in his office when he was supposed to be dead.

I was completely insulted that chemo was considered a therapy. It was obvious that the cancer wasn't killing Dad; the chemo was. My aunt, who played a huge part in helping Dad during his sickness, begged his oncologist to take him off the chemotherapy. He refused.

Dad didn't slow down for a second. He was still going to the gym every day, trading stocks, commenting on my Facebook, organizing golfing trips, planning holidays, flying across the country, scheduling my flights, calling to check in daily. My grandma often commented, "That man acts like he has no idea he's dying!"

"Let him!" I told her. "It might be the only thing keeping him alive!"

She looked at me like I'd said the first sensible thing in my whole life.

"Besides," I added, "we're all dying. None of us are facing it. All you can do is pray for him."

I was pretty sure prayer meant something different to me than it did to Grams, but I did pray for him. Every day.

Sending Light

Grandma has a saying that finally made sense to me around this time in my life. In her thick Irish accent, she'd always say, "Do the right thing, and good things will come. Do the wrong thing, and you get . . ." adorable, emphatic, dramatic pause, ". . . nothing."

I had printed out photos of my ancestors—my grandparents, their parents, and even my great-great-grandparents on my grandma's side. I framed these and put them by the window. In the morning and at night, I would light a stick of incense in front of them and say, "Love and health to my family." Then, I would send healing thoughts to Dad for a few minutes. It didn't matter how busy, tired, or disheartened I was that day. I did it with all my heart, every day, at least once.

I spent every single day revving up my prayers and my meditations for him. I'd picture a big ball of light, traveling from my little apartment in California to their house in New York. Often, I'd pictured a map, and I'd see the little light flying from Southern California to Long Island, traveling through the house, going into Dad's bedroom, and filling him up. I did the same thing for the rest of my relatives. This little light was a ball of health and wellness that I was sending to my loved ones, and even though there is no way for me to confirm if that actually worked, my dad was living much longer than a specialist had previously said he would, and he was practically pain-free.

That is, until new cancer started popping up. First in his kidney, then in his bladder, and then it spread to his lungs. His kidney was removed, and Dad was put on a different type of chemotherapy. We hoped for the best.

I thought about Grandma's advice all the time. Do the right thing, and good things will come. Good things will come. **Good things will come.**

Recovery

I was also dealing with my own recovery. Travel wreaked havoc on my progress. Even though I desperately wanted to travel, and had plans to go to London, Amsterdam, and Paris to model, I was also concerned about what that meant for my recovery. I knew I needed my herbs, practices, privacy, and comfort to keep up with my withdrawals, which were still very aggressive. A year after I had come off of every single medication I had been on since I was a kid, I was still nauseous every single day.

Every doctor I saw basically said, "Yep. You're stressed, and you're clearly going through withdrawals. Shoulda detoxed. You won't take my pills, so what do you want me to do about it?"

Little did they know that *I knew* "detoxing" in a hospital would have been terrible for my recovery. It wasn't my kind of detox. I needed to be cuddling my dog, I needed to force myself to get up to hydrate, eat well, and learn my body, I needed space to grow, and most of all, I needed to see what worked for myself, instead of having someone else tell me what worked. I knew this method wasn't for everyone, but I just said my thank-yous and walked away.

Instead of upping my drugs, I upped my meditation practices; I researched more herbs and took my health into my own hands for good. It wasn't that I didn't trust doctors, or didn't see them when I got sick, but I knew a doctor wasn't with me 24/7. I knew that regardless of a doctor's help, I had to create my own progress. I was totally done feeling helpless over my own health.

Positive Pressure

I had all kinds of pressure facing me. The word "pressure" has gotten a bit of a bad rap, I think. I had felt a fair dose of pressure in my life and had grown up quite a bit *before I had to* just to deal with it. I had created pressure for myself to change, to become better . . . but it wasn't until the pressure was positive that I ever witnessed any results. Positive pressure was different.

Positive pressure is greater than the environment that surrounds it.

Finally, I had put positive pressure on myself to get well. This pressure came from starting *My Organic Life* blog, telling everyone I met my recovery story, paying in advance for some yoga or acting classes, or whatever forced me to follow through. I was doing things that prevented me from backing out and falling short of what I wanted to accomplish. This forced me to get well and also helped me to define what wellness meant to me. I eventually created an Identity of Wellness.

Identity of Wellness

Creating an Identity of Wellness is so important because so many of us focus on our sickness instead of our health. We focus on our problems instead of our blessings. We feel envious of others instead of inspired by them. We see the bad instead of the good. When we surrender to inner guidance and our own *personal power*, instead of giving into someone else's ideas of what our wellness means to us, we open ourselves up to our *true purpose*.

This is found in something as simple as spending a few minutes a day turning off any negative self-talk and imagining your life as you want it to be. Dare to dream. **Figure out what you want.** All it takes is a few minutes of positive pressure a day.

I spent a lot of time hanging out in my meditation spot, and making plans for the future. I saw myself traveling the world, visiting places beyond my wildest dreams, completely happy. I eventually *did* go to London, Amsterdam, and Paris. I toured Italy and drove to Mexico. I flew to Florida and New Orleans and Palm Springs and Arizona. I went anywhere I could.

I even made a stop in New York before I went on my European adventures, and another stop in New York on the way back to Los Angeles. I don't think I'd ever seen my grandparents so proud. My grandma greeted me at an ungodly hour with open arms and a cup of tea, asking me how much "I fancied Europe." As European immigrants themselves, I think it meant a lot for them to see me wander around their part of the world for a few weeks.

After two weeks of wanderlust and a long bus ride from Boston to New York, then two trains and a long walk to my grandparents' home, I was safe. I slept in my childhood bed after weeks of exploring the streets of the United Kingdom and European Union, reeking of dusty museums, ancient Versailles trees, and newly absorbed experience. I had an overwhelming feeling of serene comfort when I arrived in New York, and saw the warmth of my grandparents illuminate my room.

The next morning, Dad dropped me off at La Guardia Airport for my flight to LAX. For the first time, he walked me all the way through the terminal, even introducing me to old friends he used to work with.

He was beaming.

I thanked Dad for walking me to my plane, kissed and hugged him, and watched him walk away as I waited in line for my airplane. I felt so grateful to still have him in my life I could barely contain myself. I cried grateful tears on the plane ride home, staring out the window, then called back home to New York the moment I landed to let them know I was safe.

I was back just a few weeks later, for Thanksgiving. I was happy.

The Identity Meditation

Sit with your feet planted firmly on the ground, or comfortably in lotus position.

Breathe In: I am well.

Breathe Out: I am the World.

Breathe In: I am well.

Breathe Out: I *am* the World.

Practice this for at least seven breaths. This exercise will help you feel a connectedness to your surroundings, whether you are traveling, at home, or planning to explore a new place or a brand-new phase in life.

Facing the Truth

Yogananda says in *Autobiography of a Yogi*, "Seldom do men realize how often God heeds their prayers."

Training parts of my body to align with peace, love, and the ability to deal with immense physical or emotional pain was a crucial turn on my road to happiness. Was Dad dying right before my eyes the very year I was finally getting better? Undoubtedly, *yes*. Was I going to let it interfere with my own wellness? Absolutely. Fucking. *Not*.

Sure, it made me anxious as hell. I may have even taken this out on a person or two around me from time to time, but anyone who knew I was pre-grieving—constantly waiting for the worst phone call of my life—understood my mini-outbursts. I am human, after all.

There was one strange feeling that came with those six fated months being up; Dad didn't get another diagnosis. The doctor didn't revise the original one, and say, "Okay, now you only have nine months to live." We were just waiting.

But I was grateful, above all else. Above the fear of losing him was graceful gratefulness. I was unbelievably happy that he was still here to share my life with. I was so happy that I still got to talk to him that I called. Every day. Multiple times a day, if no one answered. I always remained cheery and had good news for Dad. If nothing good had happened that week, I would just *find something*. I'd email him "10 Ways to Improve Your Golf Game" or "25 Incredible Secret Sites in Europe." He'd email me back "Photos to Take Your Breath Away" and "Amazing Landscapes." I did my best to bring my graceful grateful feeling into everything that I did. Once I saw even Dad responding to my new attitude, I got inspired to become even better. It was finally a vicious cycle of goodness, peace, and tranquility. I wasn't worried about much. I was grateful in the moment, every moment.

I was truly only worried about his compromised immune system. After Dad's kidney surgery, he had gotten a nasty case of gout. Just a few weeks later, he had resumed going to the gym every single day, using equipment that hundreds of other people were *also* using! I didn't want to discourage him from exercise, but I did encourage him to bring antibacterial wipes with him to fend disease. He was dismissive when I suggested it, but Grandma told me that he actually started to do it! Eventually, he told me that himself!

Truth enlightens people. Maybe Dad wasn't facing his death (I mean, are any of us?) but he was facing the idea of getting sick again, and I'm assuming he didn't like it.

I was also facing the truth: I was losing my dad. This wasn't just my dad, this was *Dad*, my *only* grandfather, my *adoptive* parent, and the *only* man in my life at that point who had ever shown me unconditional love, comfort, or concern. He had literally given up his entire life in pursuit of raising me, long after he was done with the idea of raising children.

That's why I think I can say that *family lies in the heart*, not in who gives birth to whom and whose name is on whose birth certificate.

Growing Up

Growing up, I showed off photos of him with Marilyn Monroe and the Beatles to my friends proudly. Because Dad couldn't carry a tune to save his life, some of my family joked that all his time around celebrities when he worked for the airlines may have rubbed off on me.

Whether Dad's time around John Lennon or Johnny Cash influenced my decision to move to Hollywood, I can't say. I can actually say it did influence *my life*.

Dad was totally obsessed with music. There was music playing in the background during the preparation of every meal. Music blared from the car every time we got in for a drive. When we first got a computer, he absolutely loved burning personal CDs and listening to them everywhere he went. He got an iPod and an iPad before I did! He *loved* technology, getting his first Facebook account at the age of seventy. He specifically loved the ability he had to customize his own playlist.

When I was growing up, Dad took a lot of comfort in deeply spiritual music, or very American country tunes. During holidays, he'd dig the '60s Christmas vinyls out from the back of the pile and put them on the vinyl player for weeks while we baked cookies and trimmed the tree. I'd sing along while we rolled cookie dough together, and he'd chime in, off-key, for the chorus. I remember opening the oven when it was taller than I was, waiting for the smell of baking chocolate chips so I could curl up to him while he read the paper in the living room. I adored my dad.

Even though I thought about these things often, they didn't make me sad. Even though I was dealing with the same old Dad, I knew he was changing every day. And I wasn't sure how long we had left together. When I had to face the idea of losing Dad, I took matters into my own hands for myself. *We're all going to lose our parents,* I reasoned, *unless we're selfish enough to want to die before them.*

I had seen how Grey's parents dealt with her suicide. Her dad carried a handkerchief around for weeks after her death, "because it's easier than tissues." He would randomly burst out crying when he spoke. No parent should ever have to go through that.

No, I was certain to be around longer than my grandparents. And, once again, I wanted to avoid illness, if I could, on the way. I was finally face-to-face with the hardest truth: I really only had myself to rely on.

Healing

I had a desire to be well *and never* get sick again if I could help it, from here on out. It was officially a year and a half since I'd quit my meds, and I hadn't had to go to the hospital once. I'd gone to get blood tests, and I'd taken doctor's suggestions for my nausea, but I hadn't filled a single prescription in that time. No trips to the ER. No prescription painkillers for my pain. No drugs for my headaches. No pills to fall asleep. No antibiotics for any cystic acne or bladder infections either. They'd both stopped completely.

My meditations worked immediately now too. I'd sit on my meditation pillow and let the ball of light pour over my whole body. Whenever I felt nausea creeping in, or an infection popping up, I pictured the warm light traveling to that spot and filling it completely until I was blinded. The nagging feelings always disappeared.

Conquering Anxiety

After self-realization, self-knowledge was my stepping stone to self-mastery. Many of my meditations consisted of just *feeling* like I was happy. I pictured my thoughts as living things, little bundles of energy. I started setting my alarm for 4:30 a.m. and taking a hot Epsom or Himalayan salt bath. In these baths, I would meditate on happiness and focus on coping with whatever life had thrown at me that week for an hour every morning, before making a smoothie, eating a raw breakfast, and taking Raelie out for a walk. With Dad's help, I had flown Raelie to California a few months after my move, and everything I did was for her as well as my own wellness. Even though I was tight for money, I desperately wanted my own space.

Soon, I was looking for a new place to live. The year lease on the apartment Raca had left me was almost up, and I was done with a studio apartment containing two people, a dog, and whatever guests I constantly let crash at the place. I spent my meditations thinking about dream houses to live in.

In my dream house, I wanted a fireplace. I wanted open windows, a bright bedroom, lots of light, a big bath, and the space for Raelie to play and run around. I wanted something entirely different than North Hollywood. I pictured white picket fences, big powerful trees, a lawn, a porch, a rocking chair, and open space. And some day, I wanted it to be close to the same beaches that Yogananda, my guruji, had walked.

After about a month of looking at apartments, I came across not an apartment, but a *house* in my price range! I couldn't believe it! It was a little north of where I currently lived, but it was still in Los Angeles, close to hiking and forests, and it had a cute little yard! I called the landlord immediately and set up an appointment at the open house.

Henry and I showed up early, and I was instantly a little deflated. Cars lined the streets, and a family was pouring out of the place. *Of course,* I thought, *it's perfect for a family.*

I paused for a moment, and let a feeling of gratitude and love overwhelm me. I took a long, deep breath and whispered, "This is my home."

I sure walked in there like it was my home! To my right was a middle-aged woman and her college-aged daughter speaking to the landlord about the neighborhood. I didn't even look their way. I scoured the house in awe. Huge, open windows! A working fireplace! A bedroom filled with light! A huge kitchen with a dishwasher! A big porch and a bathtub in a huge (twice the size of the bedroom) bathroom! A washer and dryer outside! It was exactly what I had been picturing!

And nearby? The Angeles National Forest. Free, daily, endless hiking—550,000 acres for Raelie to play and explore.

I finally met the landlord, got the tour, and thanked him with a twinkle in my eye. I was in love.

When we left, I said to Henry, "That place is mine."

He looked at me like I was being completely cocky.

"Okay . . ." he said, "I don't know. We have another place to look at today. Do you want to?"

"Let's go," I said, looking back as we pulled away. "But that place is mine."

Conviction

I had absolutely no reason to think that house would be mine.

At this point, I was living in a tiny studio apartment in Hollywood, sleeping on the same air mattress that had been left there the day I moved in. Three wear-and-tear holes had been plugged up with bubble gum. With all my travels, I had barely been home, and I was really anxious to settle down.

I was starting to think differently about everything, about who I was, what I deserved, what success meant to me. I was constantly updating these ideas. I knew weak-mindedness had led to weak actions. I was spending a lot of time in nature, taking Raelie out for long walks to the nearest dog park or hiking trail. I would turn my phone off for days. I had no one left to explain myself to. I knew who I was.

I often took Raelie to Runyon Canyon in Los Angeles, or dog-friendly trails in Malibu and Santa Monica. I'd hop on my little blue Vespa and go scooting around Beverly Hills, trying to find the best vantage for the sunset. I wandered around Melrose Place, danced under Santa Monica Pier, partied with celebrities in Beverly Hills, shared medical marijuana with wanderlust teenagers in Venice, auditioned for my first TV pilot in Hollywood, talked to the homeless, worked nonprofit gigs with the LGBT community, created a self-portrait photography series, explored an abandoned building by my apartment, took myself on dates to museums, worked on a radio show, got a residency at The House of Blues with my band, and made money on random background gigs. Just in the first few months.

I felt absolutely no pressure to impress anyone.

I was finally *free.*

The Key to Me

I was bringing myself, and also a power beyond myself, into everything that I did. I was giving this Personal Power a place in my life: to take care of things when I felt I couldn't, to give me strength when I was weak, to fix things when they were beyond my control.

You need to decide what you want to do, and then let the universe guide you to do it. You've got to interrupt your negative patterns, then allow this new positive person to *become* you, instead of striving to always become *someone.* You have to be kind to yourself, and then watch in awe as other people are more loving and receptive to you.

I let this power create opportunities for me, and I let it engage me. I felt confident that I was capable of anything I put my mind to.

I had finally recognized that the terrible, horrible, no-good person who'd been in the way all along was *Me*.

And I knew I *wasn't just* Me. Me was the ego that thought, *I want I want I want*, instead of counting its blessings. So I figured I'd give Me a backseat for a moment. There was definitely a thing beyond Me, pulling the strings. Playing the chords. Guiding Me back to the path when I ended up in the woods.

The Woods

Believe it or not, a detour or two into the woods every once in a while isn't such a bad thing. It's when we allow our consciousness to slip back into thinking of ourselves as just flesh, bones, and a body that we run into trouble, and the woods become a very dark and scary place.

The earth supplies you with everything you need to survive: it is only in our minds that scarcity lies. Most of the human race is carrying around some sort of guilt or burden that has shifted their lives tremendously from growth to stagnation. They're afraid of their Personal Power, or perhaps don't feel as though they possess it at all. As long as we define our lives by the physical, ego-driven world around us, we'll never find the answers to the deep, burning questions we're all after, such as "Why am I here?" or "What is my purpose?"

Some ways that I seek answers are really simple, everyday things that you should do to feel inspired when you are stuck. Often, when I am feeling stuck, I will go to my bookshelf and pick up a random book, open a page, and read a passage. It never matters what the book is—even some books on math or physics have always seemed to provide me with the exact answer that I need.

The Answer

I had recently picked up a Roald Dahl book, *The BFG* (short for The Big Friendly Giant)—one of my childhood favorites—at a local secondhand bookshop called Iliad in North Hollywood. I had gotten about halfway through it, and put it down for a few days to focus on researching natural ways to help Dad's cancer. I was particularly exhausted and felt very drained. Although I was grateful for every moment that I currently had with him, I was determined to find a natural path to help him through his dis-ease.

One night I had made a hot Epsom bath with flower petals for myself and picked up *The BFG* again to take my mind off of my stressful research. I got into the bath with the book and settled in, playing some soothing Eastern songs.

I got about two pages into where I had stopped previously, and my attention was drawn to something. As I turned the page, I noticed it had been bookmarked by the previous owner with a fortune-cookie fortune. As I picked it up and turned it over, I felt butterflies in my stomach.

It read simply:

Your Dearest Wish Will Come True.

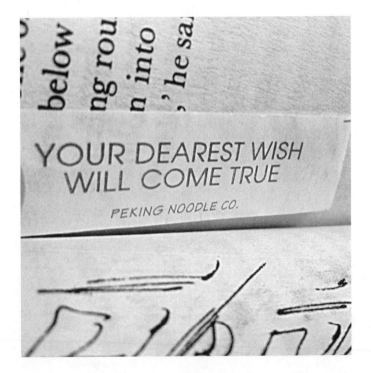

Accepting the Answer

I read the fortune over and over and over again. I paused and let it overcome me. I breathed it in and out.

It was such a powerful affirmation to me that I was on the right path that I became excited about continuing my research all over again! Not only did I finish my favorite childhood book that night, I dug deep into my wellness studies and I said a prayer to thank all of the random events that occurred for me to find that little fortune-cookie fortune when I did.

The answer never comes from just *the external*—it can't be found in another person, another book, another romp, another drink, or another party—even though moments of happiness show up in all these places. Your dearest wish *will come true*, but it can only be found *through acceptance*, and acceptance can only be found *within*.

The teacher can be you, if you choose to seek the answers, and accept them when you find them.

Accepting the answers is very difficult when you're not used to even seeing or finding them, but once you're on the correct path, they will show up for you in all kinds of unexpected and beautiful places. Keep your eyes peeled; the harder you work on yourself, the more they will guide and reassure you.

Ask yourself questions that enable you to recognize the signs that are guiding you.

10 Questions for Finding Life's Answers

1. What am I working toward at this moment?

_____

_____

2. How has finding my Personal Power benefited others?

_____

_____

3. What answers did life provide me in the past that helped me through a difficult time?

_____

_____

4. What answers did life provide me in the past that I may have missed?

_____

_____

5. How have my friends and family been my teachers?

_____

_____

6. Where is my path taking me?

_____

_____

7. Have I been leading my path or have I been led?

_____

_____

8. What events brought me right here, reading this sentence?

_____

_____

9. How can I improve myself a little bit every day?

_____

_____

10. Have I made use of all the materials provided to me?

_____

_____

You can ask yourself one or some of these questions to check yourself and create a shift in your mentality, if necessary. I constantly reference #10, because so many of us tend to focus on what we *don't* have, instead of making use of what we *do*! These answers also change over time, so feel free to reference these questions as many times a day, week, or year as you like! They're powerful tools for creating lasting change.

CHAPTER ELEVEN

DAILY MIRACLES

"Nothing is impossible. It is often merely an excuse when we say things are impossible."

—François de la Rochefoucauld (1613–1680),
French Author, Nobleman, Top-Ranking Moralist

In an instant, I had automatic emotional and physical relief at my fingertips. Everything I had was amazing, and it had been based on my life choices. It was beautiful. It was radical. It was gratifying. I enjoyed Life tremendously, not based on what I may do or what I had done: I was happy in the moment, all the time. The practices of Happiness and Health had become who I was and what I stood for. I enjoyed this security more than I had ever treasured any job, person, or material thing.

I was constantly shocked at my peaceful reactions to situations that would normally be considered stressful for others. Instead of having panic attacks or feeling completely overwhelmed, I remained calm and collected during even the most hectic situations life threw at me. It was incredibly liberating to no longer be a slave to my emotions. There was a huge difference between well-being and being well-off. I was determined to have both.

I made lists every night. I sat on my meditation pillow, took out a pen and journal, and wrote my list of activities during the day. I jotted down everything from what time I woke up to habits of personal care to what I ate and how long I had meditated. I would also write down the thoughts I had that day, especially if I was having a difficult or especially negative time.

At first, it was kind of hard. I would get Tuesday mixed up with Monday, but after a few days, I had Monday's journal entry right there, and it became easier to remember.

I made it a habit to do daily personal reflection, send light to my family, picture light within myself, and focus on my health. I made rituals out of taking my herbs, creating healthy meals, sipping my tea, listening to healing, ambient, balancing sounds, and focusing on my breath. I spent a lot more time in nature, appreciating my surroundings, listening to uplifting music, and I started exercising more. I took up a yoga practice that was personally designed to help and support my back. I took the time to think, which made me much less brash and much more kind. Friends and family started referring to me by completely different adjectives, like "kind" and "thoughtful," which were a total trip to me.

Then, I got the phone call. It was the landlord of one of the apartments I had seen, and she wanted a deposit. I hadn't heard from my Dream House yet, so Henry and I went and took another look at the apartment.

The place wasn't ideal, but it wasn't bad. Two bedrooms, a living room, a small kitchen. Not what I had pictured in any way, shape, or form, but livable until my Dream House showed up again. There was a cute record shop across the street, there were nice neighbors, and it was actually closer to Hollywood instead of farther away. I figured, *There must be a larger plan at work here.*

We told the landlord that we'd need to discuss it and would give her a deposit by the next day. It was the last month of our lease; it was go time.

We got home and got our deposit together. I was truly bummed that we'd most likely lost out on the Dream House, and I wasn't psyched about the new place, but I was totally ready to move. I drained my bank account, and started packing.

"You must do the things you think you cannot do."
—Eleanor Roosevelt (1884–1962), "First Lady of the World," Political Activist, Diplomat, Champion of Women Everywhere

Miracles

We were ready to get a new place, but it didn't exactly feel like an upgrade. I got my old, ratty suitcase out and started haphazardly throwing clothes in from my tiny hallway closet when I got a phone call.

It was the landlord from the Dream House we had seen, the house I had said "was mine" as we drove away. If we could get the deposit, the rent, and the pet deposit together by the end of the week, he said, the place was ours.

Sometimes a miracle is hearing exactly what you need to hear. I had absolutely no idea why the landlord had chosen us over families, college kids whose parents were clearly willing to pay their rent, or someone without a dog, or even why this had happened the day we were supposed to give our money over to someone else! I jumped up and down and cried tears of joy, packing with new excitement.

This was my Dream Home! And if I had gotten the call *a day later*, I would have had to say no to it because I would have given my money to someone else and settled! It came into my life exactly when I needed it, and was exactly what I had pictured, down to the bedroom with nothing but open windows all across one side of the wall. It was ethereal and beautiful and gorgeous *and it was mine*! We somehow scraped together the cash, signed the lease before the landlord could change his mind, and I was moving my stuff in before we even had electricity! I was so fulfilled, so content. I felt as though this was the first small miracle in a life that would always be filled with happy, healthy, growing miracles.

I started to make miracles happen in my daily life, instead of sitting around and wishing for them to happen. Bringing this kind of Personal Power into my life and living it every single day with such a high frequency was truly amazing.

Patience

You may be in a hurry, but Creation is not. I used to scoff at the adage "All in good time." And now I was living it happily, with exuberance, love, and excitement. They call patience a virtue for a very good reason. When I got rid of the discomfort of impatience, it was easier for me to cultivate a proper sense of how to solve everyday problems and make huge decisions for myself. I knew from withdrawals that nothing that was worth it was going to be easy, and I was totally okay with that. The payoff of a healthy mind and a healthy body was absolutely worth it to me.

Nature as Teacher

The very day I moved in, I started gardening. I was so happy to have this privilege that I went a little overboard on the plants, but I grew and nurtured each and every one from seedling to dinner table feast.

Every single morning I would get up, make a smoothie, water the plants, play hose-fight with Raelie, and check the progress of each little plant while singing to them. I loved this new ritual. It connected me to the earth and started my morning with a chore done in good fun. I also loved the progress. I really enjoyed watching my little seedlings grow into adolescent plants that soon poured out fruit, herbs, and nurturing vegetables in abundance. I loved the idea of change and growth.

There were plants I'd nurture for months and then lose to a drought or storm, but I was unaffected. I enjoyed the process of planting, gardening, and harvesting. I wasn't at all focused on the destination. It was great to eat the organic strawberries, squash, peppermint, lavender, and corn that I grew, but it wasn't quite the point.

Gardening taught me patience in a way that nothing else ever had. The longer it took for a plant, herb, or tree to bloom or flower, the happier I was with the results. I did little experiments, cloning plants and raising them in probiotic water. They grew twice as fast, naturally. I was giddy. I got to become a scientist all over again!

The therapy was in the wait. It was about forming relationships with my plants, and about understanding how much they needed from me, and what. How I behaved toward them and how much love they received absolutely affected how they grew and what crops they produced.

If you spread this theory out and apply it to your relationships with people, you can't help but see how this would have a positive effect on your life. Even applying this kind of patience, love, and understanding to yourself will have a drastic effect. It was definitely having a positive impact on my Personal Power. I was kinder and more patient; I bowed to the very power of silence.

Anger

There had been an old part of me that reveled in the idea of being angry with someone. The dislike and judgment that I had toward others had been satisfying to me.

Ask yourself, *When was the last time I was angry with someone? For what?* You may notice that a lot of the time we get angry with somebody because they believe something different than we do, or they frustrate us in some way. This is a form of im-patience.

This is also the ego talking again. Remember her? Our narcissistic friend who thinks only of "Me"? She's all kinds of real, loud and obnoxious. She's the uninvited person at the party. The embarrassing aunt at Christmas. This is where she sneaks up on us, even when we're finally cool with ourselves. It is the ego who is angry and frustrated with another person for not agreeing with us, for not being on the same page as us, or for contradicting what the ego wants us to have.

Take a breath, and ignore your ego. She's a chatterbox, and she's super unproductive for your life. Channel that feeling into something productive. Something that makes you smile and progresses your goals.

I had an especially powerful connection to myself and others when I went hiking or camping. In nature, I felt like I had finally ditched my ego for good.

"If something stops being fun, I ask why? If I can't fix it, I stop doing it."

—Richard Branson (1950–Present),
Founder of the Virgin Group and Virgin Airlines,
Humorous Billionaire, Philanthropist, Author

Becoming Who You Want to Be

As a young girl, I had always wanted to be able to spot a plant and know what kind it was. After just a few months of watching my plants grow, I could now spot many different kinds of herbs, flowers, bushes, and trees from a mile away. I took a lot of pride in knowing where in their growth cycle they were, and was always excited about sharing their unique scents and healing powers with my friends. I was becoming the girl I had always pictured I'd be. It was magical.

As I continued to practice gardening, eventually setting up a cute little upcycled path to my garden and the house, making it a new home, I lost all the satisfaction that comes with anger. Between gardening and learning more about the plants that had always intrigued me as a girl, I was provided with a new sense of satisfaction. It took on a whole new meaning.

Suddenly, being angry at anything felt *totally silly*. I knew that all I needed was in the ground, waiting to be nurtured.

Embrace the Bugs

When I was a little girl, my next-door neighbor and I played a game called Bug Island. We'd round up all the creepiest, crawliest bugs we could find and bring them to a potted plant in my front yard—Bug Island, *naturally*—and watch the bugs do their thing.

This entertained us for hours, and I swear we played this game every single day of the summer.

Anytime it rained, we would race each other outside to see who could find the most snails. We'd compare them and play with them until we were soaked. Then, we'd let them go in the dirt at the end of the day, unharmed.

Those had been my (*extremely* suburban) childhood experiences with nature, but even back then, I knew the simple fact that bugs are friends. Critters are natural, especially when you're growing your plants naturally. But when I first started gardening, I seemed to forget this. I had tested my soil, laid down new organic sod, and used GMO-free organic seeds, but I couldn't control one thing: the bugs.

They buzzed in my ears, chewed on my crops, ate up my fruit, and gnawed on my veggies. I tried every natural remedy, from using soap and vinegar water to applying beeswax to the base of my plants, but to no avail.

Once I learned to appreciate the "pests," I realized that they never actually ate any edible parts of my plants. They'd chew on some squash leaf or strawberry leaves or a part of the plant I wouldn't have used, but the edible parts—actual fruits and veggies—remained relatively untouched.

I also found my visitors totally fascinating. I would spend an entire afternoon watching ants take down a beetle and carry it back to their hole. I met many young grasshoppers, scared many lizards shitless, and even came home to some kittens that had made a home in my lavender bush. (Okay, kittens aren't exactly pests but they're still an unwelcome guest if they're using my plants as a bed! I grew them from seeds, kittens! Seeds!)

I'd find critters while I dug and happily throw them into dirtier parts of the yard where I wasn't growing. I'd let bumblebees land on my hand and I'd pet them (if you've got the nerve, they love being petted—I swear!). I noticed that the same hummingbirds would visit my garden every morning. The same squirrels came by too. This process was endlessly fascinating to me.

I also started a compost pile in my yard. Composting gives you the benefit of using every part of your plants, even if they aren't edible. Every banana peel, strawberry top, or freshly cut bag of grass went into my compost bin, giving the critters plenty of leftovers to munch on if they got hungry. The worms and maggots I found ended up here too.

Every single bee, bird, worm, opossum, raccoon, or insect I found in my yard received a warm greeting, but they never stayed for long. Nothing makes me smile more than a hummingbird in my flowers or a stray kitten lying in my lawn. And nothing probably frightens them more than a giddy young woman grinning at them from her porch.

Let It Go

Organic gardens are places of inter-being: when one element ceases to exist, it's recycled and used to create another element, allowing nature to take over in its place. I realized that even though I lived in this new, magical place, that didn't mean a host of other wildlife couldn't live here too. I was happy to share.

When I say I have an "organic garden," aside from being pesticide- and GMO-free, what I mean is that I generally do not weed. When I do weed, I either recycle the weeds to my compost, or I eat them.

I found early on that without the grass and weeds for my herbs, fruits, and veggies to lie in as they grew, much of my food would spoil before I had a chance to harvest it! It wasn't important for me to have the prettiest garden on Pinterest; it was important for me to make sure that all of my plants were interacting properly with one another, and aiding in one another's growth and progress. Let go of the idea of having a "perfect-looking" garden; instead try to focus on what the plants need to thrive.

I often planted based on which fruit I knew would need a "stern latch" to grow onto, or would need cover from the sunshine. For instance, I planted my jasmine and ivy around places, like fence posts, where I knew they would grow and thrive naturally. I let my squash grow in wads of uncut grass so it wouldn't spoil as it matured. I found this so incredibly rewarding. It was also endless, which is something else I loved.

Nature looks a certain way from afar, but once you get closer, it reveals a whole other layer of itself beneath the surface. Encounters that I once saw as a nuisance, like my daily run-ins with the critters, ended up being some of my favorite parts of my day.

My garden wasn't just mine—it was a place of inter-being that I shared with many other little creatures. Many of them relied on my garden as a food source, a shelter, or a warm place to explore their curiosities. I got dirtier, dug deeper, and became totally cool with this. Instead of trying to nitpick and force things to be perfect all the time, I was allowing nature to guide me to what was truly right and really real.

Mother Nature gives us glimpses all day long of who we really are. She invites us to connect with ourselves. She encourages us to let the small stuff go.

Treat Others the Way You Wish to Be Treated

There's no doubt that plants possess a certain kind of intelligence. That "freshly cut grass smell" that so many of us love so much is actually a chemical distress call, used by the plants to beg nearby critters to save them.

Using a laser-powered microphone, researchers at the Institute for Applied Physics at the University of Bonn in Germany picked up on sound waves produced by plants that have been cut or injured. Although these sounds are inaudible to the human ear, it was found that cucumbers scream when they are sick, and flowers let out a whine when their leaves are cut.[29]

Jesus said, "Love your neighbor as yourself." The golden rule also applies to plants. I remind myself that although I'm going to eat these plants someday, they are alive right now. I treat my plants lovingly, singing to them, watering them individually. I am extremely careful about what I nurture them with; I talk to them and I watch them grow. Because my plants interact with one another, I know that they are also interacting with and responding to me and their environment.

It has definitely made an immense difference in their growth, and taste. I enjoy hearty, healthy meals from what I grow, and I love bringing veggies straight from my garden to my kitchen to share with friends and family.

Leftovers

In the first few months I was growing over fifty different kinds of fruits, herbs, veggies, and plants. I had more food than I could actually cook or eat, and had to figure out what to do with the leftovers.

This is when I first discovered fermented veggies. You may traditionally know fermented veggies as sauerkraut, which is the most common way fermented vegetables are ingested in the United States.

Your gut literally serves as your second brain. It produces even more serotonin than your brain does! In fact, up to 95 percent of your serotonin level comes from your stomach. (When I first read that, I had to let it sink in for a moment. I mean, tell that to Seroquel!)

It's actually called your "Gut Brain" (as opposed to your "Cranial Brain") and is equipped with its own resources—breaking down, processing, and storing food nutrients endlessly without a peep. That's because the Gut Brain and the Cranial Brain are derived from the same embryological tissues and produce the same biochemical neurotransmitters that turn nerve impulses into action.

The importance of having a healthy stomach and digestive system cannot be overstated. So many issues, from anxiety, to acne, to emotional distress, to fibromyalgia, to chronic conditions, to nausea and mood disorders, can all be attributed to what kinds of foods we eat. Eating foods that seal and heal your gut is an important and vital step to staying healthy and to maintaining your health.

Your gut is also home to millions of different bacteria, both good and bad. These bacteria outnumber the cells in your body by at least ten to one, and maintaining the ideal balance of good and bad bacteria forms the foundation for good health—physical, mental, and emotional.

The Ultimate Superfood

Cultured—or fermented—vegetables are the ultimate superfood. Fermented foods are potent detoxifiers and contain much higher levels of probiotics than even probiotic supplements, making them ideal for optimizing your gut flora. In addition to helping break down and eliminate heavy metals and other toxins from your body, beneficial gut bacteria perform a number of awesome functions.

Learning about fermented vegetables was like stumbling upon the holy grail of gut wellness. For someone who suffered from chronic nausea daily, fermented foods were some of the most amazing superfoods I had discovered, and a great way to not only save the food I had grown, but heal myself as I did so! Fermented veggies helped my digestion immediately, FINALLY ridding me of frequent nausea altogether in a way nothing else had done!

In all my research, I had never discovered fermented veggies among the possible cures for my nausea. This was the icing on the cake (ironically, enough) for my wellness! Fermented veggies helped me in a way that no other drug or herb had ever helped me in the past. It drove home everything *my body* was doing for wellness. It helped my gut *process* everything it was doing, instead of constantly battling to restore its good flora in between my probiotic ingestion and kombucha drinking.

It was at this point in my life when it all finally made sense to me: my whole journey had taken me here, to this Dream Home, where I had the joy of gardening with such vigor and passion that I had extra food to ferment, to consume, and to further aid me in my continuing quest.

You've heard it before, and I'm going to tell you again: Everything happens for a reason. Everything that happens to you, every person you meet along your journey, every thought you've had all serve a greater purpose in the grand scheme of your life. Each of these little elements has something to teach us about who we are and who we are to become. Even if you may not see it or understand it at first, there is a lesson to be learned in everything we perceive as a failure or a problem. It is in learning to appreciate these little lessons that we can truly see the beauty that surrounds us, the daily miracles that fill our lives. For me, this happened in the form of playing with the critters in my garden, interacting with my beloved plants, and discovering the ultimate cure to my personal well-being—fermented food!

How to Ferment Your Veggies

If you aren't accustomed to these foods, you may have to work them into your diet gradually. Many folks like myself, who snack on them regularly, actually enjoy the taste of fermented vegetables. They have a pleasantly salty-tart flavor. Just one-quarter to one-half cup of fermented veggies per day can have dramatically beneficial impacts on your health.

WHAT YOU'LL NEED

1. Knife/grater.
2. Cutting board.

3. Your largest bowl. This bowl should be large enough to hold the entire batch of shredded veggies.
4. Mason jars are all that is necessary for both fermenting and storing the vegetables.
5. Krautpounder: This solid wood tool that looks like a small baseball bat is very handy for tightly packing the shredded veggies into your jars and eliminating air pockets. You can use a fork and your hands if you don't have one.

PREPARATION

1. SELECT YOUR VEGETABLES AND HERBS:

The first step is gathering up your veggies. Cabbage (or, as you may know it in its fermented form, sauerkraut) should be the "backbone" of your blend. Five or six medium-sized cabbages will yield ten to fourteen quart jars of fermented vegetables.

Add in hard root vegetables of your liking, such as carrots, golden beets, radishes, turnips, as well as apples, garlic, thyme, basil, celery, oregano, a pepper; just go nuts! Peel your veggies, as the skins can impart a bitter flavor. One pepper for the entire batch is plenty.

Finally, you can add sea vegetables or seaweed to increase the mineral, vitamin, and fiber content.

Once you've selected your veggies, grate them into your large bowl.

2. CULTURE AND BRINE:

For your brine, one quart of celery juice is adequate for ten to fourteen quarts of fermented veggies. While you can do wild fermentation (allowing whatever is naturally on the vegetable to take hold), this method is more time-consuming. Also the end product is less certain. Inoculating the food with a starter culture speeds up the fermentation process. You can also add the inside of encapsulated probiotics to speed up the process!

3. PACKING THE JARS:

Once you have your shredded veggies and brine mixture combined in your large bowl, tightly pack the mixture into each Mason jar, and compress using a masher to remove any air pockets. Top with a cabbage leaf, tucking it down the sides. Make sure the veggies are covered with brine and that the brine is all the way to the top of the jar, to eliminate trapped air. Put the lids on the jars loosely, as they will expand due to the gases produced in fermentation.

4. FERMENTATION:

Allow the jars to sit in a relatively warm place, such as a windowsill, facing the sun, for several days, ideally at around 72 degrees Fahrenheit. During the summer, veggies are typically done fermenting in three or four days. In the winter, they may need seven days. The only way to tell when they're done is to open up a jar and have a taste. Once you're happy with the flavor and consistency (if you've ever tasted sauerkraut this is the flavor you're going for), move the jars into your refrigerator.

For storage, refrigerating your vegetables drastically slows down the fermentation. They will keep for many months this way, continuing to mature very slowly over time.

Enjoy liberally and enjoy a cleaner gut and healthier mind!

PRO TIPS

Always use a clean spoon to take out what you're eating. Never eat out of the jar, as you will contaminate the entire batch with bacteria from your mouth.

Make sure the remaining veggies are covered with the brine solution before replacing the lid.

Living Your Truth

How much loneliness does it take to turn into cancer? How much stress does it take before someone has a heart attack? How much sadness can we endure before our bodies start to react and break down? How many pills did I need to take before enough was enough?

These are meaningless questions, because the carcinogens and dis-ease inside of us is invisible, and they appear differently in everyone. Much like these questions, most of the time a doctor cannot possibly ask us enough questions to find out *exactly* what makes a patient sick. We have so much stress, so many thoughts, ideas, actions, behaviors, and memories within a day that it would be impossible for someone else to accurately measure the exact triggers for our anxieties, fears, and health issues. Furthermore, in the first place many doctors are quick to dismiss the idea that the mind-body connection exists in any way.

Eric Cassell, a professor of physiology at Cornell, astutely pointed out that when a doctor asks her patients questions, *she's not trying to find out what's wrong with him; she's trying to find out what symptoms he might have to match classified, known diseases.*

This is an extremely important distinction.

Getting Well

I had been giving the Universe not-so-subtle cues for years that I didn't care very much about myself. I had left it up to other people not only to tell me what was wrong with me; I allowed them to define me completely based on their diagnoses. In fact, *I looked forward to the diagnosis!* It had also given me an identity and sense of self to have a label for what was wrong with me.

On the basis that something was "wrong" with me, I had taken pills for everything from ADHD, manic depression, precancerous cells, anxiety, grief, death, sadness, depressive feelings, pain, aches, and shitty life situations for almost half my life. When those pills didn't have the answers, I took different pills that promised to relieve me.

When I looked back on past experience, health issues, and the life decisions that had led up to my getting sober, I was so astounded. I looked at old photos of myself in horror; my pupils are completely dilated in every single photograph, so much so that my eye color is barely visible. My biological system was clearly working overtime to compensate for whatever was in the drugs I had taken.

What's in Rx Drugs

Pharmaceutical drugs are synthetic. They're made in a lab, and deciphering exactly what they're made from is stuff for serious chemists.

Lamictal, for example, had "worked" by blocking my sodium channels and *inhibiting* my GABA (those awesome receptors in ashwagandha, which is mentioned earlier, that work so well to keep you healthy). Lamictal blocks L-N-type and P-type calcium channels and has weak 5-HT3-receptor inhibition. *What does this all mean?*

It means Lamictal slowed down my brain. Lithium, Valium, Xanax, and Seroquel had also done this, by slowing down my GABA receptors and suppressing my central nervous system. This is where the "euphoric" feeling comes from: the drugs basically put an emergency brake on your brain activity. Keep in mind, these GABA receptors are the same ones that are so, *so* important in protecting against cancer and aiding in a healthy body and mind.

Every single drug used to treat depression, moods, and anxiety works more or less this same way. They act by out-competing the body's own neurochemicals and taking over the cells' receptor sites. Drugs like Valium and Xanax are meant to be taken short-term, but *why had I taken them, knowing they disrupted REM sleep, knowing that they were habit-forming, not knowing how they worked or what effects they were having on my body?* They hadn't come with a nutrition plan to stay healthy while I told my brain that I didn't need it to work the same way anymore! *How was this supposed to have helped me again?*

Drugs like Valium confuse the nervous system as a whole. Valium even attracts monocytes in your immune system, lowering your immunity to fight and fend off other diseases that could truly be affecting your physical body.

It was here that I realized that perhaps the purpose of pharmaceutical drugs all along was not to help me, *but to placate me into thinking I was getting well.* After all, what the pharmaceuticals were really doing was slowing down my brain. They weren't actually helping me learn to deal with any problems. This was maybe okay for people who were actually crazy, needed their brain to slow down, or had totally unmanageable lives. But what was the drugs' purpose in conjunction with talk therapy *in my own life?*

Complacent Patients

I firmly believed that many doctors would argue with me that they were doing exactly what they were taught to do when confronted with a patient like me, and I'd have to agree with that. After all, it was I who had ended up in a psychiatrist's office. That alone could confirm to the psychiatrist that I needed help, and the psychiatrist's method of help appeared in the form of psychopharmacology.

I had also taken the drugs every single day for years. What more confirmation does one need that they're necessary? They must be working, or I wouldn't be taking them. . . .

Right?

The truth was, the doctors were doing what they were supposed to be doing, and I was doing what a professional was telling me to do.

It's definitely become the norm to medicate patients in the United States. We're complacent patients, because the schooling for pharmacology is very real (and an impossibly difficult experience) so we trust the people who come out on the other side of it. We don't question what they learned because *they* don't question what they've learned.

But something didn't add up. I had gone to school for and independently learned a lot about psychology and biology. I had dozens of friends in the field! But none of us had ever been taught *any* of the natural ways of healing ourselves or our patients that I had discovered over the past year and a half!

Doesn't this seem impossibly unfair?

It only gives patients two choices: *pills, or nothing.*

Being Sick

I also realized another incredible thing at this point in my life: being sick, and being negative about being sick, *were two completely different things.*

No drug actually pairs up with a thought. There are two kinds of people: those who become defined by their illness, and those who learn from it. There's one thing I know for certain: if you don't have control over your illness, it *will* gain control over you. I met people all the time who were sick, but the difference between those who were sick and those who were living with illness was how they thought about their condition.

My friend Isabella, for example, was emailing me long diatribes about how sick and sad she was, how no one could help her, and how doctors could find nothing wrong with her besides stagnation. She begged me for help, but every solution I gave her was met with those two famous words that can bring us all down: "I can't." She had a reason why every little move toward wellness could not get done.

She was totally stuck in the past, and she constantly identified with the small diagnoses she received here and there. Finally, a doctor told Bella that based on her symptoms, it sounded like she had fibromyalgia, a word she clung to like crazy. This diagnosis completely defined her, and her sickness got worse as a result. Every time I spoke with her she was taking a new drug or doing a different treatment for her fibro, which led to other diagnoses, which required more drugs.

I didn't respond to her behavior, which surprised me. I gave her all of the advice I had, and then I took it as the warning it was.

Dad, for example, never said the word *cancer* one time. He gave it no power. He lived his life after his diagnosis as though he were cancer-free, and had already lived over twice as long as they had given him upon initial consultation. I admired this completely.

It meant that the mind-body connection was very real, not just in literature or scientific studies, but in my own life. Every single day. Much of our health and wellness is in our head, because it starts and ends there. When you truly believe something, whether it's negative or positive, your mind communicates your feelings to your body. The difference between being chronically ill and letting chronic illness define you is one thing: your beliefs.

Anything other than a totally positive outlook on life can create dis-ease. Even the smallest negative thoughts, repeated enough, stole from me. They stole my health, my ambition, my positive outlook, my loving attitude, and most importantly of all, they stole my time. There is very little in it for us. *Negative thoughts or replaying a negative memory over and over in our mind isn't helping.* In fact, *it's never helped.* Sure, you can derive a sort of pleasure—a sort of importance—by feeling like a victim or by hating someone and secretly plotting for some kind of revenge, *but really what you are doing is wasting your time and energy.*

I needed to maintain my health, all the time, at all costs. I made a list that I would read every day of the most important steps I could take to make this an everyday reality.

The Most Important Steps to Maintaining Your Health

While miracles happen every day, miracles *don't just happen.* If we don't ask for something, no one will know we need it. These same rules apply to the Universe. You need to put the work in. Miracles need to be asked for, prayed for, begged for, or we'll just plain *never recognize them.*

That's why the ancient civilizations were so enthralled by the sun. Every civilization from the Aztecs to the Buddhists to the Hindus to the Ancient Egyptians worshipped a solar deity. Mostly because it provided them with all the necessities of life—you know, the usual: food, light, and killer tans. But they also worshipped the sun because they had absolutely no idea if it was going to come up the next day.

Today, with years of science and space exploration behind us, we know that the sun's existence is a sure thing—although it *does* seem otherwise on dreary days. And if you're reading this a million zillion years from now (Hi! Is the future cool? Can we fly?!), this may not apply to you either. However, to members of these civilizations, the sun's temperamental and sometimes unpredictable behavior was a scary thought. So they prayed to it, worshipped it, and asked it to provide them with all the daily miracles of food and light. Ask and you shall receive.

The easiest way to achieve good health is to set yourself up for it. It's by recognizing those daily miracles. When something clicks for you, when synchronicity comes knocking, or when opportunity rings the doorbell, greet the moment. If your heart tells you to take a walk, take one. If it makes you happy to read your favorite book even though you just put it down, go for it. When your soul says, "Tonight, I should reach out to that friend," do it! You are a part of every sunrise, a part of the flowers blooming, and a part of the goodness of the world. The minute that those little things become your beautiful "aha!" moments, problems are much smaller and life automatically becomes more manageable.

Once I started getting up at 4:30 a.m. to meditate and watch the sun's beautiful morning dance, I saw what the ancient people were talking about—that majestic beauty that truly takes your breath away and forces you to pause for a moment. Maybe we *should* be worshipping her. I mean, *I* didn't tell her to keep rising! Did *you*?

Being Mindful

If you can move, you should consider yourself extremely lucky. I have a very dear friend named Samantha who cannot move some of her body due to a debilitating and heartbreaking illness known as muscular dystrophy. She remains one of my dearest friends and greatest personal heroines.

When I met her at the age of nineteen, she had only just then succumbed to even the idea of life in a wheelchair, after walking against doctor's orders since her diagnosis as a toddler. She finally agreed to use a wheelchair on a not-so-wheelchair-friendly college campus. We both worked to change that, and Bennington now has wheelchair access.

So, if you are able to move, move. Do something every day that gets you up and makes you feel alive. Every time I dance freely, I think of Samantha. Not in a sad way—quite the opposite. I dance for her and I think of her, because I have often danced *with* her. I've sat in her lap in her wheelchair while we rode through campus singing and screaming at the top of our lungs that the British were coming. We had fun with it.

Samantha educated me about what's possible beyond the label of "handicapped." It's incredible *what you can actually do versus what you think you can do*! So, if you can move, I say again: MOVE. It's the greatest gift you have been given.

Once I settled into my Dream House, I began to hike every single day, regardless of how sick I felt. Now that I lived just minutes from the Angeles National Forest, I was so excited about the beautiful terrain, gorgeous red sunrises, and awesome camping days that lay ahead! I connected with nature every day, every way I could.

One Thought at a Time

I remember it so vividly that I can still smell the acetone. I had been hunched over my lab desk at the scope for the eleventh hour, struggling with an equation that just didn't make sense: the asbestos levels were coming out positive, but the sample in front of me was definitely clear, meaning they should have been negative.

It was becoming clearer still that my problem was not the equation: it was my mind. I had been slipping. The long hours at the lab were a strain on my eyesight, my mental state, my emotions, my nutrition, my exhaustion levels, and my health. I had so many thoughts going through my mind at once: I was dealing with the grief of losing Grey, dealing with the breakup of my toxic relationship, I was handling the loss of many a friendship, my own health, living alone, and was still on at least ten medications for everything from moods to pain. I was struggling with consistent panic and anxiety, consumed with the fear that comes with not really knowing if what you're doing with your life is the right thing to be doing. *Worse, I carried the fear of knowing that it was exactly the wrong thing to be doing.*

I let out a long sigh, and a hand on my shoulder stopped me from closing my eyes. It was a co-worker, about to leave for the day.

"Are you almost finished?" he asked, looking at the clock. It was almost seven o'clock in the evening, and I'd been there since 6:30 a.m.

"No. I'm struggling, actually. But I'll definitely have them done by midnight." Cue a weak smile and a shrug. Try not to roll your eyes.

"Well, chill out, kid. Your mind can only hold one thought at a time."

"It feels like mine has millions at once," I replied. "But I can't hold on to any of them."

"Well," he said, "the mind can only hold one. C'mon, it's true. Try it."

I did try it, and it is true.

I thought about that encounter very often in my recovery. It was possibly one of the most important things anyone had told me before I decided to get well, because it really stuck. The mind can only hold one thought at a time. It's profound, really.

I knew that most of my thoughts had been negative, and that when my mind stopped racing for a few moments, the thoughts got depressing. When they weren't depressing, they were panicked, and when they weren't panicked, they were obsessive. That had been almost a year and a half ago. I had already come a long way.

Now, I was facing a mind that was quite the opposite. Sometimes negative thoughts would creep in, but I'd catch them immediately. I was constantly on guard at the door of my mind. I saw negative thoughts as intruders. I knew that they led to negative actions, negative behaviors, and a negative attitude. They'd been responsible for bad luck, illness, unhappiness, and exhaustion. I could only hold on to one thought, so it had to be a positive one, one that would constantly propel me forward and change me.

Does this serve me well?

Does this serve me became the one thought that truly dominated them all. It stopped the negative things from taking hold too.

If it didn't serve me, it was out of the question. Freedom and cultivating daily miracles lie in reminding yourself where your choices brought you, and what you are going to do for the future if you are in any way unsatisfied with your current life.

Pay attention to how you deal with stress. Are you taking it out on those around you, or internalizing it? Are you finding healthy ways to cope with things? Are you making time for things that make you happy? Remember, our stresses pop up physically in all kinds of different ways, from boils to tumors to nausea to gray hairs to acne to heart attacks. It's always in our best interest to confront fear and stress head-on, so that we can lay groundwork for healthy miracles to happen in our lives.

While you're practicing one thought at a time, be openminded about what you do let in, but be careful about what you let become absorbed. Think of your mind as a sponge: There are some things, like water, that flow through a sponge, even cleanse a sponge. These are your positive thoughts. But certain things, like tar, motor oil, or gasoline, will ruin the sponge forever and make it totally unusable. Think of your brain as this sponge and your negative thoughts as this tar or nasty oil. The only solution is to begin again, to start anew, and to once again go back to our "clean slate" in our meditation practices.

Recontexualizing your life—coming to a completely new idea about how it all works—is the final step to creating a healthy body that's receptive to daily miracles. This involves a certain kind of open-mindedness toward things like wellness, health, and forgiveness.

Forgiveness

I see forgiveness in two ways: as the act of forgiving, and also, as for-giving, that is, giving forth. Depending on the act, you can for-give any way you please, as long as you are bringing positive thoughts and light to the situation and begin thinking about things in a new way. This truly opened my mind up to the thought of for-giveness as a guiltless, selfless, magical thing that could do everything from soothe my worry to completely heal my relationships. For-giveness is beautiful, powerful, profound, and miraculous.

I was about to be met with the most radical kind of for-giveness of all: for-giving that which we cannot control.

Facing Fear

I did finally get the phone call I had been pre-grieving all those months, but it wasn't the one I had expected.

Grandma called to tell me that the cancer had spread to Dad's brain. There was nothing I could do, she said, so it was best I stay in Los Angeles. His emergency brain surgery was scheduled for the next morning.

Stay in Los Angeles? Oh sure, I assured her, I'll stay in Los Angeles. And I hung up the phone.

Then, I took every penny in my bank account (and some from the bank accounts of my amazing friends) and flew to NYC on a red-eye without telling my family. I called them during a layover, and informed them that I'd be there by the time he had surgery. It was too late; the oncologist had rescheduled the surgery for even earlier, and Dad was already in the middle of the operation.

When I arrived at the hospital in New York, they were wheeling Dad out of the OR and into his inpatient room. It finally occurred to me that they had removed parts of his brain in order to get the nasty tumor that had rooted in there.

Within the first hour, Dad was awake, alert, and reading the newspaper. He looked completely astonished to see me, and I saw a childlike wonder in his eyes I had never witnessed before. He discussed stocks with my family, and a part of me wondered why I had even worried. Then, the doctor came and reminded me.

My dad had a fifty-fifty chance of survival through his surgery. His blood type was so rare that they had to use a dozen donors for five pints. The tumor was so close to a major blood vessel in the brain that the odds of him not bleeding out had been another fifty-fifty. Dad had just come out of major brain surgery to remove an active tumor, and here he was, newspaper in hand!

Another crazy statistic: the tumor didn't bleed out at all. In fact, as far as the oncologist could tell, the tumor was somehow *dead*. That meant one of two things. One, that it was possible that the chemo he was taking had somehow passed Dad's blood-brain barrier and killed it, which the doctor said was highly unlikely. The other option? It just wasn't Dad's time yet. The doctor even used the word "miraculous."

Dad was never my hero more than he was in that moment, because he looked fear right in the face and didn't even flinch. Many people know fear by an acronym: *False Evidence Appearing Real*. These odds meant nothing to Dad or many people like him. Another acronym for fear is my personal favorite: *Feeling Excited And Ready*.

Facing our fears can be a powerful experience once we're ready for it. It was Osho who said,

"Suffering is not holding you. You are holding suffering. When you become good at the art of letting sufferings go, then you'll come to realize how unnecessary it was to drag those burdens along with you. You'll see that no one other than you was responsible. The truth is that existence wants your life to become a festival."

I could see now, through a combination of sobriety, hard work, love, and compassion, that suffering had not ever been holding me; I had been holding suffering.

We trust our finite, everyday experiences: the ones that allow us to drive a car, to take a test, to write a sentence, to chat with friends, to swallow a pill, to go to the beach. Those experiences are convincing enough for us to trust them, to make life-changing and real decisions by them, to base our careers or spend our hard-earned money off of them. But they're not everything.

What about the infinite connection that we constantly have to our Personal Power? The silent reverence in a memory when we smell a certain something, the excitement that gets us out of bed and working on a project we love, the feeling that makes us cry when we hear something touching, the elusive thing that makes us breathless at a lover's voice, or that makes us laugh when life is just so rough that *it has to be humorous*? Where is the time allocated to appreciate *those* daily miracles?

Mainstream psychology and a lot of holistic books like to point out that many sick people "need" their sickness. Psychiatry points the finger at itself, saying that chronic illness is a form of self-punishment, revenge, or a deep feeling of worthlessness. I will not argue against these insights, except to suggest that *they may be harmful to the healing process.*

I know at my sickest, *it would have really hurt me personally to hear that I was making myself sick.* Sure, I had co-created my illness, but getting better does not happen in a moment, even if you want it to. Sickness had been holding me back from absolutely everything in life: I could barely get out of bed to run to the bathroom *to get* sick, never mind any thought process that went along with ever feeling healed. Sure, I had done it to myself, but *the idea that I was still doing this to myself was absolutely absurd.*

Was the argument *really* that everyone on earth who gets sick makes themselves sick? Everyone on earth gives themselves cancer and nausea and migraines and suicidal thoughts and heart attacks? Every tumor ever diagnosed and every ingrown hair and every ulcer is self-caused? Every single dis-ease-caused death was that person's fault?

Well, no. It's a lot more beautiful than that.

Beauty

Okay, let's back up and begin with our good friend, DNA, the building blocks of your cells. Your DNA knows exactly what information to pick out and how it goes together for everything it "says" chemically. That is how you exist, right now, reading this. Besides building and rebuilding itself constantly, DNA knows how to build RNA (ribonucleic acid), its counterpart and nearly identical twin.

RNA's life goal is to travel away from DNA in order to produce proteins (more than two million that we know of). These proteins naturally repair the body. They are the genetic masters of our health. RNA strands are continuously made, broken down, and reused. RNA is responsible for the transference of genetic information, while DNA is responsible for the long-term, silent storage of it.

This is where it gets interesting.

Only 2 percent of the genetic material in DNA is used for complicated coding, self-repair, and manufacture in RNA. That leaves 98 percent of RNA doing absolutely nothing that science can account for, except that we know it is synthesized when DNA is needed.[30]

The Encyclopedia of DNA Elements (ENCODE) project suggested in September 2012 that over 80 percent of DNA in the human genome—non-coding DNA, it's been termed (it's worth a Google)—"serves some purpose, biochemically speaking." *They just don't know what that purpose is.*

This non-coding DNA is turned into functioning RNA molecules. I believe that the purpose of this non-coding DNA— in humans, we can't account for the activity of as high as 98 percent—is used for maintaining our health. This is a small part of where our Personal Power lies. This is what gets us up when we feel we cannot move, this is what allows people to miraculously cure themselves from cancer or other harmful, fatal illnesses. Our bodies are biologically predisposed toward health and wellness. I think that health lies in the silent moments between ego-driven life. When the body is silent, comforted, and rested, it can repair, heal dis-ease, stay young, rejuvenate, and recover.

This has immense implications about exactly how tremendously capable we are of healing ourselves. We've already covered that a doctor cannot possibly ask enough questions to find out exactly what makes us sick. We know that our bodies and nature have internal analogues to all the drugs that we take for most pain, and all depression, anxiety, and mood swings. We've covered that your thoughts have biological consequences, based on your emotional awareness, and thinking good thoughts, eating clean food, and meditating on your goals have a real, scientifically proven result.

A cell, when it talks to the rest of the body, is not unlike the brain. It correlates millions of messages, and has other messengers within it to carry out chemical exchanges that must "keep up" with themselves every second. In fact, *a cell is more active than the brain is because it never "sleeps."*

Those who will mindlessly watch their own cut heal and think nothing of it are doing themselves a grave disservice. They will just as easily dismiss people who recover "miraculously" from cancer and other chronic illnesses by means of strict lifestyle change and earnest meditation, not understanding how beautiful it is that every time you get a scratch, infection, or bruise, *your body recovers from it without you even having to consciously do anything.*

Reaction

We were born to react. When we get into heated debates with our loved ones, when there's competition, when we hear something nasty about ourselves, when we fight with family, the ideal thing we want to do is get into a movie-style debate and respond, "Oh yeah? Well, I can be crueler/meaner/more threatening." When a loved one says something that hurts, it's very tempting to dwell on it, where it came from, why it happened. What a waste of time, eh? I mean, we're talking *family*. Will we ever figure those people out?!

The nerve impulse for worry often shows up in the body as an ulcer in the stomach, as a spasm in your body, or in your muscles as a knot. Sometimes it shows up in your head as a migraine, but every cell in the body remembers it, which triggers chronic illness. You may even consciously forget that you are worrying, but the body never forgets. When the feeling comes back to the body it may as well never have left.

To bring yourself back to your true state, remember that you must relax your body and mind to release your health and let your body do the work.

Get Real

Let's be real. Sometimes we don't have time to lie down or chill out during stressful moments and do these super helpful exercises. But taking at least a few minutes of your day to notice what's good about your life and how you're caring for yourself will change you instantly for the better. This, in itself, is a self-loving action. Taking this time not only brings miracles forward in your mind, it attracts them. That is why constantly being present, aware, and vigilant about recognizing daily miracles as a part of your life is essential.

If you're spending time with someone whom a doctor said should be dead, if you hear good news when you're down, if a stranger says just what you need to hear, if you get your dream job or your dream house just as you were ready to settle, congratulations! You've found your daily miracle.

Meditation to Bring Yourself Back to True State

Sit up straight in a seat or on the floor with your palms facing upward.

Take a deep breath through your nose, and let it out through your mouth.

Think of your cells going to work in your body, repairing, renewing, replacing old, broken-down parts of you that are no longer serving you. Release what is no longer serving you, accepting what is new as light.

Breathe In: "The little cells are drinking."

Breathe Out: "The little cells all are thinking."

Breathe In: "I welcome wellness to step forward."

Breathe Out: "I invite wellness into my home."

Breathe In: "I choose Light."

Breathe Out: "I release Fear."

Continue this meditation until you can see and *feel* your cells going to work repairing your body. This little meditation will help connect you to daily miracles and enable you to start creating the life you truly desire.

CHAPTER TWELVE

LIFELONG HEALING

"In meeting yourself, free of all shoulds and musts and wills, for even a moment, you realize that even if nothing gets fixed or done, simple natural fulfillment is already here."
— Gangaji (1942–Still Kickin' It), Spiritual Teacher, Author, Nonprofit Founder, Radical Peacemaker

Cultivating healthy habits is one of the biggest steps to true, lifelong, natural fulfillment. Tony Robbins said, "Human history is basically the history of human belief." You are, essentially, living in a room you've built yourself based on the foundation of your beliefs. A sick mind in a healthy body, or a healthy body in a sick mind, just aren't compatible.

We get so wrapped up in either dwelling on the past, or being apprehensive about the future, that we forget to be grateful and present. Happiness is not an ever-elusive thing that you need to strive for constantly. It is a muscle, a habit, a living thing, and there are ways to grow it and nurture it, the way you would a plant. Earnestly practicing even a handful of these habits I've mentioned in this book will be sure to make you a happier, healthier person!

The simplest and most important things that you can do for yourself is to treat yourself naturally and with forgiveness. The stigma of depression, the fear of inadequacy, and the lethargy of unhappiness can often get in the way of recovery. Managing symptoms of depression or dis-ease requires a practical, proactive, and peaceful approach to counteract anxiety and fear.

Being Brave

What is fear, really? It's a belief. A belief that something will cause you harm, a belief that you're not good enough, a belief that the unknown is frightening. Fear is always going to be there—it's a biological necessity, a survival instinct. Every person reacts differently to different situations. There is not a magic recipe for managing your fears, but there is a guidebook.

The hard truth is, people lie. They get confused. They're subject to human error. They're fallible. The last time someone projected their shit onto you is—I can guarantee you—not the last time someone will. The idea is to figure out how to handle these things so that they don't trigger us. As real as your emotions feel to you, finding a way to check yourself and remember that you have control over them—and not them over you—is essential to finding positive and peaceful solutions to these never-ending issues and problems.

My dear friend Nicole got pregnant last year. A few months ago she gave birth to a beautiful baby boy who wasn't breathing properly. They still don't know why, but just twenty-three hours after his birth, baby Ryaan died in Nicole's arms. She and her husband were completely devastated. They never got a chance to bring Ryaan home from the hospital.

Nic shared a post on her Facebook page that we can all take a lesson from. She wrote:

> I've been going through so many highs and lows on this roller-coaster ride of grief. A couple weeks ago I decided when I was in a good place to write a letter to myself to remind me of some realizations. Here's what my letter to me, from me, says:
>
> Dear Nicole,
> There are no mistakes. There's nothing extra, nothing less. There are no "shouldn't haves." All the people you

meet, all the events in your life, good, bad, or otherwise, are unfolding as part of a perfect and unfathomably complex whole.

It's like building a puzzle without the image on the box; you put the pieces together as they seem to fit but you can't see the bigger picture. You get a sense of the colors and textures, but don't really know what it is you are creating. Yet you know that each piece has its place.

Likewise, this moment is just as fleeting as the blink of an eye, a sliver in time; but never once doubt that are you anywhere but exactly where you need to be. *Even at the lowest low, so deep in despair that you believe there really is no way out, remind yourself that not for a moment is your struggle futile; not for a moment does what you are feeling or experiencing have no place. It is an intrinsic part of the whole.*

Remember that the mere ability to FEEL the depths of your emotions is pure beauty, pure potential. To feel great sorrow is a sign that you are more than able to feel great joy. When you deny, avoid, or neglect intense emotion, out of fear that you are not strong enough to make it out the other side, you do yourself a great disservice. You cannot block the pain and let in all the joy. We don't get to pick and choose. It's all or nothing.

After all, if you decided to toss out all the ugly pieces, how would you ever get a glimpse of the whole and beautiful picture?

Love,
Nicole

The first step to making this transformation permanent is to start by making a decision. You have to decide to be brave, coura-geous, and audacious. Decide that fear is not going to control you. See tragedy as an opportunity to grow. See it as an oppor-tunity to do more, become more, and succeed more. Without beliefs that motivate us, we're left completely disempowered. Nicole and her husband are happily pregnant with Ryaan's little sister. While she says a part of her was terrified at first, she knows that she's already experienced the greatest tragedy and she knows what to do with herself now when she sees it. I also have this confidence, having faced my own disempowering thoughts and beliefs head-on.

Every fear faced is another roadblock that you've overcome, another step toward the future of your dreams and the Story of Your Success.

The Story of Your Success

You aren't here to shrink away from your desires; you're here to pursue them. Do what feels right for you in the pursuit of your dreams today, especially if it feels out of your comfort zone. Send that email to the company you've always wanted to work for! Sign up for that yoga class you've always wanted to take! Start the first chapter of that book you always wanted to write! Whatever gets you over the hump, make it into a beautiful ritual that you look forward to every day. Directing and bringing forth this passion every single day is the key to everlasting change.

Practice For-Giveness

Let go. For-give yourself first, and then forgive others. Whenever I have a less-than-pleasant thought about something or someone, instead of ruminating about the thoughts, I start a brand-new mantra.

I start by saying, in my mind, "Love to" whomever. So, for instance, if Joe Derp has cut me off in traffic, instead of cursing him out, I say (sometimes out loud), "Love to Joe Derp." This helps a lot. It refocuses me and I can concentrate on for-giveness. I for-give Love to Joe Derp, instead of im-patience and rage.

Whatever works for you to get you unstuck from this bloody cycle of holding on to things—do it. Because you only have one life, and it's yours alone. Holding on to grudges or being cynical about others isn't helping anyone—especially not you! It's only wasting your time and distracting you from powerful creative goals and pursuits.

Listen Up

Communication is the key to every relationship, especially your relationship with yourself. Ultimately, listening will be the key that unlocks the door to your happiness. Part of communication is more than speaking your mind.

Listen first. Seek to understand. Then, with the information that you have gathered, you can form a conclusion and finally let all your thoughts out if need be. Or y'know, just lock that mouth up and throw away the key!

Sometimes other people need an ear so they can vent, they need a soundboard, or they need to get out ideas. Your opinion is valued much more highly when you listen first and speak second. This one took me a very long time to learn, but I have to say at this point I consider myself a pretty excellent listener, and I've gotten very good at keeping quiet when I have nothing to say. What I've learned from other people when I stopped to listen has been much more remarkable than anything I did or said while running my own mouth!

There are people who say you have to do things a certain way: some people think you should go to church every Sunday, others may think you should go to work every weekday from nine to five. Other people might be fallible, and subject to human error, but their opinions are always worthwhile, and can be endlessly fascinating if you choose to see them that way instead of always waiting for your turn to speak.

"Plenty of people miss their share of happiness, not because they never found it, but because they didn't stop to enjoy it."
—William Feather (1889–1981),
Publisher, Author, Lover of Swanky Bow Ties

Smile More

Smiling more—even a forced smile—has been proven for decades to make you happier. Smiling helps to prevent us from looking tired, worn down, and overwhelmed. When you are stressed, take time to put on a smile, or even laugh out loud—even if it's a forced laugh! Stress should be reduced and you'll be better able to take action.

Smiling is absolutely free. And smiles let the world know you're happy. Studies have shown there is a measurable reduction in your blood pressure; smiling releases endorphins, natural pain-killers, and serotonin.[31] This makes smiling a natural drug.

Seeing videos of myself when I was practicing for acting auditions in LA was revealing. Often, when I spoke, the corner of my mouth turned down instead of up, as if I was frowning in between words. Not cute! I started smiling, even when I was sad. I made it a daily habit. I didn't want a trace of a disappointed life reflected in my face, and other people responded immediately. I made nicer friends. I got cast in sweeter roles. I was actually genuinely happier about everything I did. Smiling conjured up joy inside of me. Instead of waiting for happiness to happen, I was bringing happiness into everything I did.

A big smile is my favorite greeting, and the one I always remember other people by the most.

Facing the Truth

It wasn't until two brain surgeries later that Dad started having serious complications. The oncologist had decided that brain radiation was Dad's best option for beating the cancer. Other than nausea and a lack of taste, he wasn't complaining too much from the radiation sessions. Then again, he wasn't one to complain. Even when he was limping, Dad would insist he was fine. We all believed him, but photographs don't lie. His beaming, perfect smile slowly turned into a noticeably forced smile that was clearly hiding a deep grimace.

I visited New York as much as I could, but I was becoming concerned about the steroids they had Dad on for the brain inflammation. I was getting excited phone calls from him at odd hours, and I wasn't sure what to make of them. Anytime I told him I might not be home the next month, the calls got more excited and frantic. Then he'd book a plane for me. Every six weeks, like clockwork. This type of behavior was like dealing with a different person.

When I confided to Grams about this, she admitted that he'd been different.

"Different how?" I asked.

"I don't know," she whispered, and I could hear her checking the adjoining rooms to make sure he wasn't around. "We don't even really talk anymore."

It was hard to hear her heartbreak. They'd been married for fifty-six years.

Then, he started to fall. By the time I came home for Thanksgiving 2013, Dad had a walker. Every morning, and every night, we carried him up and down the stairs to his office, or outside to the car. He could no longer drive, but he didn't want to sign his car over to anyone.

"What about when I get better?" he asked us.

What could we say?

I had all the hope that Dad did. I was convinced that his condition was temporary, and that he'd recover. I sent light to him every morning and night. I meditated on his health. I gave him all the healthy advice I knew, and educated myself every single day ferociously. I did physical therapy exercises with him at home, stretching his muscles for him to use and move his feet, holding him to walk. I encouraged him to drink caffeine-free tea, made him as many superfood, probiotic-based meals as I could, forced water on him, and said a lot of prayers.

When I came home for Christmas, Dad was in a wheelchair, and his body had become frail. I wondered when the change in his attitude had happened, because he no longer seemed excited or enthusiastic about recovery as he had when I was home for Thanksgiving just three weeks before.

Then, my grandma told me, "The doctor told him he'll never walk again."

This was the crippling blow. Not the cancer. Not the pain. Not removing his kidney, parts of his brain, or giving him brain radiation. Not the chemo. Not even the paralysis itself. No, the end came when my dad succumbed to the idea that he'd never use his legs again.

My dad, who took me on a mile walk and then a three-mile run every single night, would never golf, drive, go to the gym, or run again, and he finally believed it. Belief is funny that way. This was the same man who had completed every NYC Marathon since the first one in 1970 until retirement age. The same man who was going to the gym just weeks after brain surgery. A man who kept a logbook of his physical activities—every single day—since the 1960s. He even wrote an entry the day I was born. He had managed to get a run in.

I was on a plane back to New York less than a month and a half later, to visit Dad in hospice. By the time I arrived, he was completely unconscious, breathing shallowly, and I could feel that it was his last few hours in his body.

I held his hands and said a lot to him, but I knew he'd never say another word to me again.

His nurses all said he was waiting for me to come home to pass. I said my good-byes, called my family to come, and at 4:19 a.m. on February 19, 2014, Dad took his last breath in a room full of his loved ones.

Those last sleepless eleven hours by my dad's side, watching him struggle to let go of his life, remain some of my most burdening and most cherished memories of my time on earth thus far. I felt completely helpless, and yet completely at peace for him once he finally passed away.

I realized, suddenly, that I had not ever actually pictured the day that he'd die. And here I was, fatherless, at twenty-seven. Again.

Once Dad died, a part of me felt like I had been robbed. The thoughts of, *This isn't fair at all. What am I going to do? What am I going to do?* plagued me every day from the night I saw him pass away until many weeks after the funeral. Grief has a funny way of sneaking up and robbing us of our clearer mental faculties. I really just couldn't believe that he was truly gone. I was devastated and fearful all over again.

Life's Interruption

The day after Dad's funeral, I got up early after unsuccessfully trying to sleep in my childhood playroom. It had been raining all night. In fact, the day of the funeral had been the foggiest, coldest, hardest downpour New York had seen in years. We couldn't even bury him, it was raining so hard, and as I put the last flower on my dad's casket without seeing it go into the ground, a part of me had felt a surreal distance from the closure I had expected. It wasn't a movie-style funeral. We didn't stand by his gravesite as they lowered him. We didn't throw any dirt over him. We just drove away.

As the sun came up, I went to Dad's bedroom. I buried myself in his covers, drinking up his smell. I opened his closet, went through all his drawers, and read everything he'd written. I traced his hand-writing with my fingers, I dug my face deep into his pillows. I discovered his running journals, dated since 1975. I looked over the framed photos, including one of us together when I was five.

I threw on a sweater, a scarf, and a big coat, shook my boots free of last night's rain, pinned my headphones to my ears, turned on some music, and headed out to get a bite to eat.

It slowly occurred to me on the way to the deli that I had not said anything to anyone since the night before, and had no idea if I could even speak. I was so deeply buried in the last few hours; I had gotten on a plane, gone to hospice, watched Dad die, spent two days at the wake and a day at the funeral, and had woken up after sleeping barely a wink. I was fighting some major nausea, and felt a sincere emptiness that only a bare house the day after a funeral can evoke.

As I headed to the deli, headphones on max, I almost turned around. *How can I ever speak to anyone again? How can I decide what to eat? How can I read a menu? How can I make a decision? How can I eat, how can I go on? What am I supposed to do now? What if someone asks why I'm in town? I don't think I can say another pleasant word to—*

Just then, a man across the street caught my eye. It was still so early that the streets were mostly empty, and he was pointing and shouting. I took one headphone off and he was muffled. I cocked my head, made a super confused face, and almost moved on, but he shouted louder, determined to get the message to me.

"At least it's not raining!" he yelled, smiling and pointing to the sky.

It took me a second to process. At. Least. It's. Not. Raining. I looked up suddenly at clear, blue skies. Off to my right, the sun was penetrating golden hues through stubborn clouds. It was beautiful.

Right! At least it's not raining!

I smiled back, "I know, right?"

The words escaped my lips with a slight rasp, but I surprised myself with a sincere chuckle. He nodded and pleasantly moved on.

That was the first time I thanked Dad for interfering with my fearful thoughts. *Of course I could talk to other people! Of course I could go on, move on, eat, make decisions, take a flight back home, work, and live again! It would suck for a while, it would be hard, and I wasn't sure what the next moment would look like, but it wasn't hopeless.*

And hey—*at least it wasn't raining!*
I drank in the sun and walked into the deli.

Facing Your Fears for Good

It takes a while to adjust to losing a parent, a child, a relative, a significant other, or someone very close to us. And there is no timeline for this kind of grief. It is totally okay to be so dumbstruck by the fact the person who raised you, who you raised or intended to raise, or someone who loved you dearly is not around, that you are paralyzed.

I walked around in a grief cloud for weeks. I woke up crying hysterically from dreams where Dad was alive, for months. I didn't want to be awake because I thought of him, and I didn't want to sleep because I thought of him. Perfectly normal.

I could grieve in a healthy way, but I didn't want grief to ruin my life. I could miss him, but I needed to *cherish him* instead of letting The Missing take me down. I knew that the last thing Dad would want me to do in this situation would be to cave, flail, or fail. After a few weeks of facing the idea of life without him, I began consciously replacing all my fearful thoughts with a new mantra: *How Can I Make This Good?*

Instead of fearing life without Dad, I tried to see him in the little things around me, as well as the big. Every time something good happened, I thanked him. Every moment of life that synched up, I gave Dad a silent high five. There were days I would be walking and crying, and I'd feel him with me.

Although it was comforting to feel him everywhere, it truly wasn't the same as him being alive. I was still bitter, angry, and felt very lonely. All the thoughts that I had as a kid of life possibly not getting better, of my grandparents dying before everyone else's parents, and of ultimately being left alone surfaced all over again. I had to fight these thoughts constantly, while also dealing with the other effects of grief, a job, and day-to-day stress.

Then, I had a dream. I was backstage in the auditorium in which I grew up doing shows, right across the street from my childhood home. It was a stage my grandparents had seen me on plenty of times.

I was so incredibly nervous because someone had mixed up the costumes. I was supposed to be wearing a black costume and mine was pink—the jokes wouldn't make any sense this way! I was totally panicked and my heart was racing.

As I was arguing with someone on the crew, the curtains came up suddenly, and I immediately broke out into song. As I looked out into the packed audience, everyone was silhouetted, including my grandma. Everyone except for Dad, who was lit up in a bright light, sitting in the middle row with a big smile on his face and applauding loudly.

That dream was the most beautiful confirmation to me that Dad still has my back, and is always cheering me on, even when I am freaking out, having a bad day, or feeling totally alone. I am so grateful he showed up this way, and continues to show up every day.

Honestly, I feel him in this reassuring way all the time; when I'm struggling, when I'm confused, or when I'm lost, this proud, smiling version of Dad always shows up in someone or something. And I am always so happy that I know how to recognize him.

Get Grateful

The most important way of dealing with grief or a traumatic experience of any kind is to get grateful. This is actually just a matter of switching your language until you're done accepting these super-disempowering thoughts into your life. The bare basics are simple. Just spin every negative thought you have into a more empowering and positive new one. I know it sounds too good to be true, but some of life's toughest questions have simple answers that would amaze you, and this happens to be one of them. When practiced earnestly, it will give you immediate results! Let me give you a few examples of some Old Thoughts that I had, and the New Thoughts that I replaced them with. I didn't just read or vaguely understand these New Thoughts, as we so often do. I truly felt, applied, and experienced them.

Old Thought: I've only had twenty-seven years with my Dad! This is unfair!
New Thought: I deeply cherish the twenty-seven beautiful years I got to spend with this amazing, selfless man who loved me every way he knew how. How lucky I was to get twenty-seven (not one or two but twenty-seven!) full, lovely years with my grandfather!

Old Thought: How could a doctor take Dad's hope like that? How is cancer still killing people? What kind of special interest is involved if they're poisoning people with the cure?
New Thought: What can I do to be proactive about other people's recovery from this kind of experience? How can I help the next person go through this in a positive way? How can I educate myself about this subject?

Old Thought: Life is unfair! I am alone and I have no support.
New Thought: This situation has presented me with an amazing opportunity for growth and a chance to find out who I am without relying on anyone else's approval or support. This will give me an empowered sense of self and accelerate the growth of my Personal Power.

Old Thought: No one will ever understand my hurt!
New Thought: Many people have experienced grief, sadness, and great pain throughout all of history. How can I learn about how those people have dealt with their experiences positively, to serve themselves or others? How can I bring a light to this that no one may have shed before, in order to help others overcome their hurt?

Old Thought: No one cares that this traumatic experience happened to me!

New Thought: Everyone is fighting a silent battle I may know nothing about. It is my duty to treat others with a smile, kindness, and respect, regardless of how I am feeling, because they may be hurting too. This will allow me to experience new opportunities that I may have closed the door to in my grief.

Old Thought: I am fearful of losing everybody that I let myself love.

New Thought: The capacity to love is a gift. The ability to go on, day in and day out, after feeling sadness is also a gift. I have felt joy as well as sadness, and will feel joy again. If I can get through this, I can get through anything. I have all of the tools I need inside my own mind to cope with any loss that comes my way.

Practicing even some of these thought-changing techniques will give you a better grasp of your awareness and gratitude, and make your problems much more manageable.

Dreams

Not long before Dad passed, synchronicity found me again. This was totally random. I went to San Diego to meet a friend, and suddenly found myself coming off the train in the town of Encinitas and facing, of all places, Swami's beach. The beach where Yogananda had written *Autobiography of a Yogi*.

I walked the two blocks to Swami's and the Self-Realization Fellowship in a dreamlike state. Not only was the view absolutely breathtaking, I had found the foundation! The Foundation of Yogananda's fellowship, and the foundation of why I had packed up and moved out to California to begin with!

Swami's beach is gorgeous—clear waters reflect a perfect, aqua blue sky with white sand and a breathtaking view of the Self-Realization Temple and Cardiff's weathered cliffs. Palm trees line the streets and silhouette the perfect landscape. The beach is mostly empty save for dedicated runners, sandy surfers, and quiet yogis. An occasional baby seal will find his way onto dry land lined with flocks of seasonal seagulls. I could visit the Self-Realization Temple and Meditation Gardens daily with a short walk from the train. This kind of synchronization was appearing everywhere, and made me happy despite losing Dad. I felt so grateful that my dreams were really coming true.

I've walked Swami's beach many times. I went there the last time I spoke to Dad on the phone, and I headed there after I arrived back in California from the funeral. I've written almost every page of this book at Swami's. I have gone there many times to think, meditate, practice yoga, watch the sunset, talk with friends, surf, run, and walk Raelie on the beach. There, I feel a connection to Yogananda, to Dad, and to myself. It's a connection that I haven't found anywhere else.

I still have my Dream House in LA, but I also have a new house. There's a white picket fence, huge, open windows, space for Raelie to run around, and a beach view of Swami's and The Self-Realization Temple. I walk the same beaches as my guruji daily. I meditate on the shores and listen patiently in Yogananda's meditation gardens for my Personal Power to speak to me.

All because I let myself take a train once to meet a new friend.

Back to Basics

I purchased health insurance for the first time just a few weeks after Dad passed (thanks, Obama!). The first time I saw a doctor after Dad died, I told her I was grieving, and she suggested antidepressants. I had no idea *how I hadn't seen this coming.*

"A good friend of mine just lost her mom," she said, getting out a prescription pad, "and they really helped her. I mean, don't get me wrong. They're not magic. They're not the solution, but they did help my friend a lot. Let me get you a small dose; you don't have to—"

"No, thank you," I said, almost automatically, "I don't take it."

She looked at me inquisitively. "Don't take what?"

Uh, I guess I hadn't thought about that in a while.

"I don't take antidepressants or mood stabilizers or pills of any kind like that," I replied, adding, "sorry."

"Oh. Oh! Okay, okay, yes. You don't take medicine? I may need to prescribe you medicine to help you!" she said, jotting it down.

"I take medication if I need to. I just don't take psychopharma."

"I see, I see," she said, writing in the margins, but crossing nothing out. Making fierce eye contact, she asked, "So, what drugs were you addicted to?"

"Oh, no. I wasn't addicted to . . . I mean. No drug problems. I just don't take it." I smiled pleasantly.

"They're not harmful," she said, and assured me that if I ever changed my mind, I could tell her.

I promised I would.

It could have all ended right there. It was as easy as saying yes, or even suggesting something I had been prescribed before. It would have taken nothing more than identifying with previously being diagnosed with a mental illness. It would have taken nothing more than getting and filling that prescription, to go back to where I was three years ago. One nod and I could have gone straight back to relying on whatever pill I wanted to numb me out, using Dad's death as the excuse that no one could argue with.

Saying no felt incredibly rewarding. Of course no one would blame me for wanting to cover up my feelings, *but I didn't want to cover them up. I wanted to deal with them.*

Dealing

The words "I can't deal" used to fly out of my mouth countless times a day. Even faced with the most deeply penetrating grief of my life, I never let this sentence even enter my mind.

Less than a month after Dad passed, I was wandering around Expo West: The Natural Products Expo in Long Beach, California, working for one of my favorite all-natural products companies and seeing everything as if for the first time. Grieving at home, alone, was not my thing, and I felt no pressure to do anything except to experience the moments I was in.

I checked in with my ego all the time, but she was actually going through grief the same way that I was. Moving on in this way wasn't about *getting over it*. Instead of thinking about Dad as gone, I thought about him as just passing on to a different form. One that I could allow to positively affect my life. This honestly came *from* feeling him everywhere—not the other way around. I accepted it gratefully.

I was gathering a whole new perspective of myself, especially now that I knew and could feel that Dad was on my side. He was doing things in death he was never able to do in life.

For instance, once I opened myself up to working through my grief, opportunities came my way like rapid-fire. My acting career accelerated overnight, and I found myself working beside some of my favorite artists and actors. This included many artists whose music had helped me along my journey, including Young Money, Arctic Monkeys, Selena Gomez, and Jason Mraz. I worked on *Ted 2* with Seth MacFarlane (we even snapped a few pictures together!), the creator of *Family Guy*, a show that I had turned on so many times to "make myself laugh" when I was most hopeless. Now he was my boss.

I was hired by some of the companies that had propelled me on my green beauty journey, becoming the face of La Bella Figura's new organic makeup line. I traveled to New Orleans to do a photo shoot with the founder, which was a dream come true. I started working directly for major all-natural brands that I had only once coveted. Delizioso Skincare, one of the first brands that I had switched to in my early natural beauty days, approached me about creating a collaborative organic and natural makeup and skin care collection.

TARA: The Glow Collection by Delizioso Skincare is vegan, all-natural, organic, and getting more loving feedback every day. We launched it on the one-year anniversary of Dad's passing. Our products have bases of the organic oils that most changed and saved my life, like argan oil, Barbary fig seed oil, and jojoba oil. Five percent of our profits go to the Cancer Research Institute, in honor of Dad.

Getting Guided

After Dad's death, I continued to feel guided by his presence. I asked for daily miracles, I left myself open to them, and they were coming straight to me. I was led to every single book I needed to read, every single person I needed to talk to, and every quiet or awakening moment I needed to have. Facing my fears was having some awesome results. I was manifesting everything I wanted.

I found myself working with the same people whom I had only once admired, and becoming friends with people who had propelled me to where I was: my life was aligning, and everything was coming full circle.

Practically everything I ever wanted Dad to see me accomplish has happened after he died. This could have made me extremely bitter, but instead, it made me very proud, and determined to do even better. I knew Dad had a hand in all of this goodness in my life, and even though a part of me was sad he wasn't here to see it "in person," another big, grateful, happy part of me knew that he was watching every step peacefully, applauding with a big smile from a bright place.

Two Doves in a Cherry Tree

"A man is like two doves in a cherry tree. One bird is eating the fruit while the other silently looks on."

—Ancient Indian Proverb

There are two parts to you: the part that does the action, and the part that watches you do it. As you read this, there is a part of you that's reading, and there is a part of you that's watching you read. It's breathing your breath, it's keeping your posture, it might even be turning your pages.

To cure anxiety, to fight depression, to beat illness, and to get control of ourselves, there is another layer to transcend, all of which happens in the gaps where you are reading this—thinking, reading, breathing, talking, digesting, and so on happen *above* the experience of real life. We may say we are reading, but the study of how these words will affect our body in the future is something we have little knowledge of. This seems a little impossible to study, but it's beautiful and quite easy to study in ourselves.

You needn't go anywhere special to find your truth: only "back" to the beginning. You need to wake up. Many things "out there" exist, but we haven't been trained to observe or see them.

When Raelie growls at something I don't see, I may say, "Hey! Stop that!" But I *do* know that she perceives something, hears something, maybe, that I am not aware of. I sometimes forget that this is why humans bred dogs—to protect us. If it was thousands of years ago, her growl may have encouraged me to take lifesaving action. In fact, today, it still might, if I'm aware enough to notice.

We appear to have all the channels, but apparently we're stuck on three—waking, sleeping, and dreaming. For instance, to see what your sleep is like, you'd have to be awake, watching yourself sleeping. To see how you have truly shaped your own life, you need to turn on your Consciousness and observe it. Without guilt, without fear, and without judgment. Once you can observe yourself awake, you will realize that life is just a beautiful, grand dream.

Curing Ourselves

When you're sick, you go to a doctor and say, "I am sick, please cure me!" But when you cure yourself, you don't go to a doctor and say, "LOOK! I am cured!" At least, you're not encouraged to, because we casually assume that the person who cures herself naturally, who survives a disease, or who overcomes a dis-ease is made of different mental or physical machinery than the rest of us.

They're not. This mental machinery and chemical outline are the same for you as they are for anyone else, but the mental process can be large or small. Earnest meditation, good habits, positive thoughts, and getting grateful all teach us to control the process that is constantly, consistently influencing us every day, whether we realize it or not.

Almost none of the successful people whom you know of started out that way. Richard Branson was broke at the age of forty, with Virgin Airlines and Virgin Music under his belt. Gandhi was a selfish, disgruntled lawyer when he started helping people. Benjamin Franklin was in so much debt by the time he got to America that most of his diaries are just wishes and prayers that his collectors stayed at bay. Lucille Ball grew up on stage with Ginger Rogers and let Paramount starve her and shave her eyebrows off before she struck out on her own. Ball was forty before *I Love Lucy* hit the air. Obama was a funny-looking mixed kid with an absentee dad. No one knew his name outside of Chicago until he was forty-six years old. Dolly Parton grew up on a cow farm. Thomas Edison failed a thousand times before his lightbulb actually lit up. The list goes on and on. . . .

We live in an incredibly open and diverse world. Facebook, the largest social network, creates no content. Uber, the largest taxi service, owns no cabs. Airbnb currently the largest accommodation provider, owns no hotels. eBay, the largest online trade retailer, carries no inventory.

It's never too late to become a meaningful specific, live your dreams, or jump-start your life. Your own limitation is your imagination.

The Lifesaving Meditation

Get in touch with yourself today.

Take five minutes to spend quiet time writing your goals, learning yourself, opening your mind to new methods of food preparation or different healing techniques, and becoming aware. Free-write your thoughts lucidly right now. Jot them down in the margins if you run out of room here. Better yet, start a brand-new journal!

Try to write for an hour every single day. If you feel that you cannot find time to do this, cut out something else you do that may not be serving you. For example, watching TV or sleeping for an extra hour. Meditation and goal-writing can be more helpful in naturally relaxing and focusing us than sleep or "zoning out."

It certainly can't hurt you to learn YOU. Take this book as another powerful tool on your journey. I am still happily, and with wide eyes, going through mine. Open it to any page, any day, and take your lesson. The worst thing that can happen to you is that you never strive for anything better than what you're currently doing—even if you're a millionaire, or completely content.

There's a reason why some people who become millionaires— even billionaires—are still miserable. They compare themselves to others, they try to please other people, they live in a sea of negativity and in a cage of monotony, or they spend too much time focusing on either their past or their future.

I wasn't forced to change; I was compelled to change. The very environment I lived in compelled me to change, and Love guided the way. Love got me here. Love is the reason I survive, and belief in Love is the reason I thrive. The only reason that I not only survived, but happily thrived, through grief, pain, and withdrawals in the last three and a half years was because I had faith in myself and faith that the Universe had bigger, better plans than I did. Nothing more. The Universe has constantly confirmed this to me in both large and small ways, each and every day. I hope I have helped confirm it to you.

One Thought

As I conclude this book, I've read and reread the chapters preceding this one over and over again, and one thought continues to strike me: "I do not remember writing *so much* of this!" In the space where writing was taking place, my Personal Power, the part that was healing my skin, breathing my breath, and growing my nails, was also whispering to me in the background. I was being guided every step of the way. This is when words, actions, and thoughtful habits flow out of us and things start to really fall into place.

You can learn by trial-and-error experience, or you can learn from the mistakes others have made. That is why I am so ferocious about reading books and furthering my education. It's selfish and altruistic all at once. I want to make my own life better, but I want to make others' lives better too, before they're at their wit's end, before they're sick and tired of being sick and tired, and before we lose another beautiful soul going through a hard time. I know that troubled souls on depressive paths can be rerouted, and can use their lives to make the world a better place. I am living proof.

I hope that after you put this book down, you feel like you can act to make your life better, and you can start working on your dearest dreams and deepest goals. I hope that you begin to access your Personal Power. That is my greatest hope for you.

There is no substitute for taking loving action. Approach your day pleasantly, and with Self-Love. Promote yourself and your well-being first, and the rest will take care of itself. You can positively affect and change your own life immediately. I wish you all the luck and love in the world.

And remember: you can only focus on one thought at a time.

So make it a good one.

NOTES

1. Ellen Jean Hirst, "Pharmacy sales boost Walgreen earnings; CEO says goodbye," *Chicago* Tribune, December 23, 2014, http://www.chicagotribune.com/business/ct-walgreens-earnings-1224-biz-20141223-story.html; Reuters, "UPDATE 1-Strong prescription sales help Walgreen top profit estimates," December 23, 2014, http://www.reuters.com/article/2014/12/23/walgreenresults-idUSL3N0U730920141223.
2. Dr. Henry K. Beecher, "Ethics and Clinical Research," *The New England Journal of Medicine* 274, no. 24 (1966): 367, http://www.hhs.gov/ohrp/archive/documents/BeecherArticle.pdf.
3. F. Gstirner and H. H. Kind, "Chemical and physiologic studies of preparations of valerian," *Pharmazie* 6, no. 2 (1951): 57-63.
4. P. Olivier, R. H. Fontaine, G. Loron, J. Van Steenwinckel, V. Biran, et al., "Melatonin promotes oligodendroglial maturation of injured white matter in neonatal rats," PLoS One 4, no. 9 (2009): e7128. DOI: 10.1371/journal.pone.0007128.
5. M. F.P. Peres, E. Zukerman, F. da Cunha Tanuri, F. R. Moreira, and J. Cipolla-Neto, "Melatonin, 3 mg, is effective for migraine prevention," *Neurology* 63, no. 4 (August 24, 2004), http://www.neurology.org/content/63/4/757; Natasha Turner, "5 benefits of melatonin beyond a good night's sleep," *Chatelaine*, September 5, 2014, http://www.chatelaine.com/health/wellness/five-surprising-benefits-of-melatonin-that-have-little-to-do-with-sleep.
6. K. B. Alstadhaug, F. Odeh, R. Salvesen, and S. I. Bekkelund, "Prophylaxis of migraine with melatonin: a randomized controlled trial," *Neurology* 75, no. 17 (2010): 1527-1532. DOI: 10.1212/WNL.0b013e3181f9618c.
7. R. D. Altman and K. C. Marcussen, "Effects of a ginger extract on knee pain in patients with osteoarthritis," *Arthritis and Rheumatism* 44, no. 11 (Nov 2011): 2531-8, http://www.ncbi.nlm.nih.gov/pubmed/11710709.
8. K. C. Srivastava and T. Mustafa, "Ginger (Zingiber officinale) in rheumatism and musculoskeletal disorders," *Medical Hypotheses* 39, no. 4 (1992): 342-8.
9. V.K. Goud, K. Polasa, and K. Krishnawamy, "Effect of turmeric on xenobiotic metabolizing enzymes," *Plant Foods for Human Nutrition* 44 (1993): 87-92.
10. K. Linde, M. M. Berner, and Kriston, "St. John's wort for major depression," Cochrane Database of Systematic Reviews 4, no. CD000448 (2008). DOI: 10.1002/14651858.CD000448.pub3.
11. K. Linde et al., "St. John's wort for depression—an overview and meta-analysis of randomised clinical trials," *British Medical Journal* 313 (1996): 253. DOI: http://dx.doi.org/10.1136/bmj.313.7052.253.
12. Richard P. Brown, Patricia L. Gerbarg, and Zakir Ramazanov, "Rhodiola rosea: A Phytomedicinal Overview," *HerbalGram* 56 (2002): 40-52, http://cms.herbalgram.org/herbalgram/issue56/article2333.html.
13. Carolyn Cidis Meltzer, Gwenn Smith, et al., "Reduced Binding of [F]altanserin to serotonin type 2A receptors in aging: persistence of effect after partial volume correction," *Brain Research* 813 (1998): 167-171.
14. Y. H. Qiu, X. Y. Wu, H. Xu, and D. Sackett, "Neuroimaging study of placebo analgesia in humans," *Neuroscience Bulletin* 25: 5 (2009): 277-82. DOI: 10.1007/s12264-009-0907-2.
15. C. Galesanu and V. Mocanu, "Vitamin d deficiency and the clinical consequences," *Revista Medico-Chirurgicala a Societatii de Medici si Naturalisti din Iasi* 119, no. 2 (2015): 310-8.

16. Mike Adams, "Popular Shampoos Contain Toxic Chemicals Linked to Nerve Damage," *Natural News*, January 11, 2005, http://www.naturalnews.com/003210.html#; MSDS Data Sheet for Sodium Lauryl Sulfate; MSDS Data Sheet for Sodium Laureth Sulfate; AScribe Newswire, "OCA & Cancer Prevention Coalition Warn of Hidden Carcinogens in Baby Care," Feb 28, 2007; *Technical Evaluation Report: Sodium Lauryl Sulfate*, prepared by ICF Consulting for the USDA National Organic Program, February 10, 2006; http://www.ewg.org/skindeep.

17. Agency for Toxic Substances and Disease Registry (ATSDR), "Toxicological profile for aluminum," (Atlanta, GA: U.S. Department of Health and Human Services, Public Health Service, 2009). http://www.atsdr.cdc.gov/toxprofiles/tp22.pdf.

18. "Chemicals Known to the State to Cause Cancer or Reproductive Toxicity," last modified January 3, 2014, http://oehha.ca.gov/prop65/prop65_list/files/P65single01032014.pdf; Rhodes MC., et al., "Carcinogenesis studies of benzophenone in rats and mice," *Food Chem Toxicol* 45, no. 5 (2007): 843-851; International Agency for Research on Cancer, "Benzophenone," 2012, http://monographs.iarc.fr/ENG/Monographs/vol101/mono101-007.pdf July 1, 2014; E. Mikamo, et al., "Endocrine disruptors induce cytochrome P450 by affecting transcriptional regulation via pregame X receptor," *Toxicology and Applied Pharmacology* 193, no. 1 (2003): 66-72; G. Kerdivel, et al., "Estrogenic potency of benzophenone UV filters in breast cancer cells: proliferative and transcriptional activity substantiated by docking analysis," *PLoS One* 8, no. 4 (2013): e60567; Y. Nakagawa and K. Tayama, "Estrogenic potency of benzophenone and its metabolites in juvenile female rats," *Molecular Toxicology* 75 (2001): 74-79.

19. National Toxicology Program, "Report on Carcinogens, Twelfth Edition. Butylated Hydroxyanisole," (2011). Environmental Working Group, "Butylated Hydroxytoluene," *Skin Deep*, http://www.ewg.org/skindeep/ingredient/700741/BHT/; Environmental Working Group, "Butylated Hydroxyanisole," *Skin Deep*, http://www.ewg.org/skindeep/ingredient/700740/BHA/; V. Labrador et al., "Cytotoxicity of butylated hydroxyanisole in Vero cells," *Cell Biology and Toxicology* 23, no. 3 (2007): 189-99; R. S. Lanigan and T. A. Yamarik, "Final report on the safety of assessment of BHT (1)," *International Journal of Toxicology* 21, no. Suppl 2 (2002): 19-94; S. H. Jeong et al., "Effects of butylated hydroxyanisole on the development and functions of reproductive system in rats," *Toxicology* 208, no. 1 (2005): 49-62; T. Masui et al., "Sequential changes of the forestomach of F344 rats, Syrian golden hamsters, and B6C3F1 mice treated with butylated hydroxyanisole," *Japanese Journal of Cancer Research* 77, no. 11 (1986): 1083-90; A. A. Botterweck, "Intake of butylated hydroxyanisole and butylated hydroxytoluene and stomach cancer risk: results from analyses in the Netherlands Cohort Study," *Food and Chemical Toxicology* 38, no. 7 (2000): 599-605.

20. P. D. Darbre, A. Aljarrah, W. R. Miller, N. G. Coldham, M. J. Sauer, and G. S. Pope, "Concentrations of parabens in human breast tumours," *Jounral of Applied Toxicology* 24, no. 1 (Jan-Feb 2004): 5-13.

21. C. P. Marston, C. Pereira, J. Ferguson, K. Fischer, O. Hedstrom, W. M. Dashwood, and W. M. Baird, "Effect of a complex environmental mixture from coal tar containing polycyclic aromatic hydrocarbons (PAH) on the tumor initiation, PAH–DNA binding and metabolic activation of carcinogenic PAH in mouse epidermis," *Carcinogenesis* 22, no. 7 (2001): 1077-1086; Ministry of Healtth, Labour and Welfare, "Standards for Cosmetics," (2000), http://www.mhlw.go.jp/english/dl/cosmetics.pdf (accessed July 23, 2014); European Commission, "Crude and refined coal tars," *CosIng*, http://ec.europa.eu/consumers/cosmetics/cosing/index.cfm?fuseaction=search.details&id=28255 (accessed July 23, 2014); European Commission, "Chromium trioxide," *CosIng*, http://ec.europa.eu/consumers/cosmetics/cosing/index.cfm?fuseaction=search.details_v2&id=28884 (accessed July 23, 2014); European Commission, "Cadmium and its compounds," *CosIng*, http://ec.europa.eu/consumers/cosmetics/cosing/index.

cfm?fuseaction=search.details_v2&id=29456 (accessed July 23, 2014); European Commission, "Arsenic," *CosIng*, http://ec.europa.eu/consumers/cosmetics/cosing/index. cfm?fuseaction=search.details_v2&id=28880 (accessed July 23, 2014); "IARC mission," International Agency for Research on Cancer (IARC), accessed July 31, 2014, http://www.iarc.fr/en/about/index.php; International Agency for Research on Cancer, "Agents classified by the IARC monographs, volumes 1-109," accessed July 31, 2014, http://monographs.iarc.fr/ENG/Classification.

22. C. J. Edmonds, R. Crombie and M. R. Gardner, "Subjective thirst moderates changes in speed of responding associated with water consumption," *Frontiers in Human Neuroscience* 7, no. 363 (2013). DOI: 10.3389/fnhum.2013.00363.

23. http://theorganiclifeblog.com/tara-mackey-ogles-osmia.

24. American Academy of Clinical Toxicology and European Association of Poisons Centres and Clinical Toxicologists, "Position paper: ingle-dose activated charcoal," *Clinical Toxicology* 43 (2005): 61–87.

25. Amy Larocca, "Liquid Gold in Morocco," *New York Times*, November 18, 2007, http://www.nytimes.com/2007/11/18/travel/tmagazine/14get-sourcing-caps.html.

26. H. Bennani, A. Drissi, F. Giton F, L. Kheuang, J. Fiet, A. Adlouni, "Antiproliferative effect of polyphenols and sterols of virgin argan oil on human prostate cancer cell lines," *Cancer Detect Prev.* 31, no. 1 (2007): 64-9; S. Sour, M. Belarbi, N. Sari, C. H. Benammar, C. H. Baghdad, F. Visioli, "Argan oil reduces, in rats, the high fat diet-induced metabolic effects of obesity," *Nutr Metab Cardiovasc Dis.* 25, no. 4 (April 2015): 382-7. DOI: 10.1016/j.numecd.2015.01.001; K. Q. Boucetta, Z. Charrouf, H. Aguenaou, A. Derouiche, and Y. Bensouda, "The effect of dietary and/or cosmetic argan oil on postmenopausal skin elasticity," *Clin Interv Aging* 10 (2015): 339-49. doi: 10.2147/CIA. S71684.

27. Q. Fang, C. Huang, C. You, and S. Ma, "Opuntia extract reduces scar formation in rabbit ear model: a randomized controlled study," *The International Journal of Lower Extremity Wounds*, epub ahead of print (2015 Aug 27), pii: 1534734615598064; T. Nakahara, C. Mitoma et al., Antioxidant Opuntia ficus-indica extract activates AHR-NRF2 signaling and upregulates filaggrin and loricrin expression in human keratinocytes," *Journal of Medicinal Food* 18, no. 10 (Oct 2015): 1143-9. DOI: 10.1089/jmf.2014.3396.

28. P. Leevutinun, P. Krisadaphong, A. Petsom, "Clinical evaluation of Gac extract (Momordica cochinchinensis) in an antiwrinkle cream formulation," *Journal of Cosmetic Science* 66, no. 3 (May-Jun 2015): 175-87; G. P. Sidgwick, D. McGeorge, A. Bayat, "A comprehensive evidence-based review on the role of topicals and dressings in the management of skin scarring," *Archives of Dermatological Research* 307, no. 6 (Aug 2015): 461-77. DOI: 10.1007/s00403-015-1572-0.

29. Peter Tompkins and Christopher Bird, *The Secret Life of Plants* (New York: Harper & Row, 1973); Omer Falik, Yonat Mordoch, Lydia Quansah, Aaron Fait, and Ariel Novoplansky, "Rumor has it...: relay communication of stress cues in plants," PLoS One 6, no. 11 (November 2, 2011): e23625. DOI: 10.1371/journal.pone.0023625.

30. "Noncoding DNA," *Wikipedia, The Free Encyclopedia*, https://en.wikipedia.org/wiki/Noncoding_DNA.

31. J. D. Laird, "Self-attribution of emotion: the effects of expressive behavior on the quality of emotional experience," *Journal of Personality and Social Psychology* 29, no. 4 (April 1974): 475-86.